# The Abortion Myth

Leslie Cannold

•

# THE ABORTION MYTH

•

*Feminism, Morality, and the Hard Choices Women Make*

•

*WESLEYAN UNIVERSITY PRESS*

*Published by University Press of New England*

*Hanover and London*

Wesleyan University Press
Published by University Press of New England, Hanover, NH 03755
©1998 by Leslie Cannold

Introduction, Appendix, and Bibliography
©2000 by Leslie Cannold

Foreword ©2000 by Rene Denfeld

Original Australian edition published in paperback by
Allen & Unwin, St. Leonards, NSW, 1998.

Library of Congress Cataloging-in-Publication Data
Cannold, Leslie.
    The abortion myth : feminism, morality, and the hard choices women
make / Leslie Cannold.
        p.    cm.
    Includes bibliographical references and index.
    ISBN 0–8195–6377–3 (alk. paper).
    1. Abortion—Moral and ethical aspects.   2. Abortion—Public
opinion.   3. Women—Attitudes.   4. Feminism.   I. Title.
HQ767.15.C38    2000
363.46—dc21                                                    99–34374

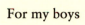

For my boys

It does not follow from the feminist position that holds that only a pregnant woman can decide about abortion that abortion raises no moral issues.

—ROSALIND PETCHESKY[1]

She is caught between her own perception that the abortion was a responsible decision and the conventional interpretation of abortion as a selfish choice.

—CAROL GILLIGAN[2]

Moral responsibility in pregnancy . . . involves a responsibility not just to maintaining the existence of the fetus, nor even just a commitment to providing the care and nurturance needed for it to flourish, but a commitment to bringing into existence a future child. My claim is that the decision to abort is a decision, for whatever reason, that one is not prepared to bring such a child into existence.

—CATRIONA MACKENZIE[3]

To be a mother is to take on one of the most emotionally and intellectually demanding, exasperating, strenuous, anxiety-arousing and deeply satisfying tasks that any human being can undertake. It is a task that shapes and changes you so that you see yourself, and other people see you, in a different way. It also entails commitment that, in one form or another, lasts for life.

—SHEILA KITZINGER[4]

# Contents

# Foreword

## Rene Denfeld

Several years ago, a friend of mine was considering having an abortion. She is one of many women who are adamantly pro-choice but say they could never have an abortion themselves. Now, thanks to a broken condom, she was in what she called a family way. She was also underemployed, single, and living in a tiny studio apartment. It was not time for a child.

It was that phrase "family way" that stopped her in midsentence. She explained to me that she had always planned on a family, but not alone. In her value system, it was important to have a partner for raising a family, and important to have a steady income. Even more important was an emotional readiness for the trials of parenthood. "I don't have the patience for children yet," she said. Finally she confessed, "I don't think I would be a good mother right now."

The decision my friend had to make was a moral decision. It wasn't about abstract issues of personal rights or her own desires. It was about her view of right and wrong, including the right time to have a child. Above all, it was about the importance of being a good mother.

This conversation came back to me reading *The Abortion Myth*. Leslie Cannold spoke to everyday women who support abortion, and to those who do not. She began with the assumption that we are all moral people, whether we defend the environment or put loggers first; whether we fight racism or repeal affirmative action; and whether we believe in protecting the unborn or protecting abortion rights. That we have rights does not remove the moral considerations that come with them.

Cannold posed difficult ethical scenarios for the women. Would you abort if you knew the child could be adopted? What if the fetus could be raised artificially? Is it morally okay to abort for a personal reason, such as, if you were offered the honor of a trip to attend the Olympics?

What Cannold discovered was that those who support abortion rights and those who hate them agree on one important issue: abortion involves making moral decisions. Even women who wholeheartedly support the right to choose take into account women's motives in choosing abortion: Did she think it through? Has she weighed her options carefully? How women feel about abortion is often decided by how much they trust other women to make this moral choice.

The women who aborted in Cannold's study were not flippant or selfish about their choice. Like my friend, they believed in family planning. They wanted their children to enter a family that was ready for them. They wanted their children to be loved and well cared for. They knew parenting is hard work and a serious responsibility. And they felt their decision was not just best for themselves, but for their future children. In short, women who abort are not only making a moral choice, they are often making a good moral choice.

As Cannold writes, women kill their fetuses because they care.

• • •

For feminists who preach non-violence, abortion poses difficult ethical questions. If killing is wrong, what is abortion? Arguments that the fetus is not alive and that abortion therefore is not "killing" strike many women as disingenuous. That is exactly why women have abortions: in order to kill a fetus that will otherwise develop into a child.

But does the death of a fetus mean that abortion is an immoral choice? Life is full of hard, sometimes tragic choices, decisions that we may not be altogether comfortable with. We might have to put an elderly parent in a home. We might have to take our husbands or partners off life support following a terrible car accident. That we grieve our decisions does not make them wrong.

Our choices as parents are especially powerful, even life-deciding. We can immunize our babies, or risk exposing them to serious illnesses. We can use modern medicine to reduce a fever, or we can use prayer, or herbs. We can spank children for punishment, and no state will interfere as long as we don't leave bruises. We can decide if our children should pray nightly to Jesus, or honor the Goddess. We can even teach our children to hate those we hate.

The women in Cannold's study spoke of abortion in terms of the complex responsibilities of motherhood. As she writes, women who abort are making not just "a decision to end a pregnancy, but a decision not to become a mother." It is motherhood, chosen or imposed, that is central to the abortion debate.

Yet the rights and responsibilities of motherhood have been largely ignored on both sides of the politicized abortion debate. As much as the women in Cannold's book disagree on abortion, they tend to agree on the importance of motherhood. Motherhood, Cannold tells us, is the common ground on which a more complex understanding of abortion can occur.

· · ·

Why has the morality of abortion been so silenced? We have ethical discussions about other tough reproductive issues, such as egg donations, surrogate parenting, or fertility drugs that produce octuplets. Rather than resulting in efforts to outlaw such practices, open public discussion has sometimes expanded their acceptance. In the least, it has created understanding for the women and men who make such choices, such as the parents in surrogate cases.

When morality gets raised in terms of abortion, however, it is invariably in an attempt to limit its legality or availability. This has made many feminists rather tentative about the topic.

As a result, feminists have largely avoided the moral question and stuck to arguing personal rights to defend abortion: the right for women to control their bodies, the right to choice, the right to medical privacy. In fact, abortion has been portrayed as so private it cannot even be talked about. We publicly hash out the ethics of assisted suicide but shout "hands off my uterus!" when confronted with abortion.

As Cannold details, the personal rights argument has reduced abortion to a battle: woman versus fetus. In order to argue that the rights of a woman are paramount, feminists have had to argue that the rights of the fetus are irrelevant, that it has no value, that the fetus is no different than a scrap of tissue. And so feminism has found itself depicting pregnancy as akin to having a bad case of warts. Such a cavalier attitude toward pregnancy and motherhood does little to enhance either abortion rights or respect for the importance of parenting.

It also plays directly into the hands of those who would paint feminists as baby-killers. The right wing has grabbed the moral high ground, depicting abortion as selfish murder and the women who have them as immoral, heartless souls. Pro-choice advocates have found themselves on the defensive, backing up at every turn while the anti-abortionists advance, using their moral shears to prune the "right" of abortion down to the ground. In the United States, women in rural areas too often have to drive hundreds of miles to get an abortion, provided they can find the transportation. Clinics are segregated from other medical care and vulnerable to assault. Women who have agonized over whether to abort find themselves running a gauntlet of committed believers.

•   •   •

Cannold makes it clear that morality is not a side issue or a new political slogan for abortion rights. It is a crucial concern during a time when technology is rapidly changing the nature of reproduction. Already, women advertise their eggs to the highest bidder; we can test fetuses for birth defects and terminate those who will be disabled; gender selection is on the table, and "customizing" your infant's hair color, personality and other attributes may be on the way. Brain-dead pregnant women are being held on life support, simply so they can deliver a baby. And the point of fetal viability keeps getting earlier.

In coming years, we will wrestle with difficult questions about the ethics of reproduction, and abortion will be central to the debate. If a fetus can be easily removed and gestated, will the window of time in which a woman can have an abortion keep shrinking until the procedure is entirely illegal? Will courts be able to take an endangered fetus away from its drug addicted mother? Can an unborn fetus be a ward of the court and put up for adoption? Will life be defined by the economic worth of a fetus, making white fetuses more valued than black or brown?

These questions are going to land like a bomb on top of abortion rights, and we had better be prepared.

• • •

Those of us who support abortion would do well to heed Cannold's advice, and develop a moral defense of women who abort. We need to stop dissecting women into wombs and fetuses, and recognize their hearts as well as their rights. Above all, we need to trust that given such a weighty responsibility, most women (and men) pursue a moral decision with the utmost care and concern, just as we do in other trying circumstances.

My friend did decide to have an abortion. She mourned for that baby, and she saw it as a baby, for some time. Eventually she met the person she wanted to be with, and her plans for a family came true. Today they have a child. She says she doesn't regret her abortion. She doesn't think about who that child might have been. She is comfortable that as its mother she made the right choice. It was a moral choice.

# Preface

One half of all pregnancies in the United States and England are unplanned. Unplanned pregnancies account for two out of every three pregnancies in Australia. In the United States every year, 3 percent of women aged fifteen through forty-four have an abortion. Australian, English, and American women make a lot of decisions about pregnancy and motherhood during the course of their reproductive lives. This book explains how they manage the moral complexity of these decisions.

Received wisdom about the morality of abortion has it that, at best, abortion is the lesser of two "evils," or an unavoidable "sin." Yet what many women know is that sometimes abortion is not the *most* moral choice, it is the *only* one. Anti-choice supporters tend to put a lot of energy into "proving" that the fetus is "alive." They assume that success on this front will lead to their audience agreeing with their two other (implied) points: that abortion is killing, and that killing is always wrong. University of Notre Dame ethicist Janet Smith, for example, claims that women "having abortions are killing their own babies . . . a woman who states that she thinks abortion is killing is . . . acting in violation of her own [moral] principles when she opts for abortion."[1] A recent speech by a conservative New York senator put it more baldly: "Ladies and gentlemen, we all know that abortion stills a beating heart."

Recently, however, pro-choice supporters have realized that proving the fetus is alive and that abortion kills it does not prove that abortion is wrong. Pro-choice Australian writer Karen Kissane, says that "any woman who has felt a baby stir inside her [and] any man who has seen the tiny heart pulsing on an ultrasound screen, knows that abortion is about ending a life."[2]

British abortion activist Eileen Fairweather also points out that "one Australian study [found] 60% of women believe life begins at conception (compared with 36% of men). That doesn't stop [women] having abortions . . . It is possible for people to support a woman's right to choose whether they believe abortion is killing or not."[3]

The women I interviewed, no matter what side of the abortion fence they were on, were clear that the fetus is alive, and abortion kills it. None of them, however, believed these facts proved that abortion was wrong. They argued that the relationship pregnancy creates between themselves and their fetuses makes it both necessary and right that they had the power to make such life-and-death decisions. For these women, the central moral issue was whether or not a woman's decision to abort was—or was not—justified. What differentiated a choice to "kill from care" and an immoral abortion choice was the pregnant woman's motives, behavior, emotions, and decision-making process. Did she have good reasons? Did she consider everyone's needs and interests? Did she make her decision thoughtfully and lovingly? Grieve over the need to make the decision at all?

Most of all, for abortion to be a moral choice, the pregnant woman needed to think of herself *as* a pregnant woman, to consider the mesh of interests that spring from the utterly unique relationship between herself and the could-be child within her. Adoption was consistently rejected by the women I spoke with as an irresponsible way of coping with an unwanted pregnancy, because of the pain it would cause the mother in the short term, and the child in the longer term. Charity's choice to abort her pregnancy is a good example of "killing from care":[4]

My decision to have an abortion was a decision I made to care for the child that was within me. To adopt that child would be more cruel to me than just ending it, because it's giving the child no help. It's saying "Well, it's not my problem." My decision to abort will affect my child in a humane manner, because I've got my child's interests at heart. That's why I decided to terminate, for that child's sake.

For a myriad of complex reasons, most feminists have strenuously resisted seeing abortion as a moral issue. A Marie Stopes International abortion counselor quoted in a recent book on abortion insisted that:

The idea that we all suffer to some degree when we decide to have an abortion makes me furious, because it's not true. Most women do not experience any guilt, remorse or doubt . . . I see very few people who actually have a moral qualm about abortion itself . . . at least 90% of women feel no ambivalence about abortion. For most, it's a very straightforward practical decision.[5]

The few feminists who have agreed that abortion is a moral issue have been reluctant either to suggest ethical standards against which women should be judged or to actually pass anything other than neutral or laudatory judgments on the abortion decisions women make. Part of the feminist reluctance to discuss abortion morality derives from their overall feminist skittishness about discussing the flipside of rights: responsibilities. A recent clipping in the news section of *Ms.* magazine, for example, questions the feminist credentials of a male academic who argued that men might be more comfortable with the increase in women's rights if they were accompanied by an increase in female responsibility:

### CALL IRON JOHN!

This just in from the *Chronicle of Higher Education*: Bryant College professor Harsh K. Luthar . . . claims that because most studies on sexual harassment are written by women, men are getting paranoid: "This includes both male managers and professionals, many of whom live in a nonclinical but nevertheless unnatural state of paranoia in light of the changing legal and societal expectations that impose on males increased responsibilities for social sexual interpersonal relations without any parallel increase in responsibilities for female workers, professionals, and managers."[6]

The results of my research provided absolutely no support to feminists arguing the "abortion is straightforward" line. The women I interviewed were clear that abortion was a difficult *and* a moral decision. In the same way, these women didn't shirk from making a less than laudatory appraisal of a particular woman's abortion decision, or in making the larger judgment that women's responsibilities in the abortion decision are just as important as their rights. Almost all the women I interviewed saw the abortion issue as revolving around the pregnant woman's decision-making process. An abortion decision that did not reflect a woman's "feelings" and "love" for her could-be child and other significant people in her life, and that was not motivated by care and protective concern for all those she loves, was just plain wrong. An example of a woman who deliberately conceived and then aborted, for instance, was roundly condemned by almost all the research participants for lacking the required feelings about conception, pregnancy, the fetus, and motherhood. Pro-choice Gillian had straightforward views on the matter: When you terminate, "you're thinking of yourself and you're thinking about the baby. It's not a cold decision. But getting pregnant in order to kill the baby! Doing it intentionally just doesn't seem right. Having a baby to kill it, there's no you in that. You're just setting out to murder, [to commit] premeditated murder."

Again, unlike the few feminist forays into abortion morality, the women I interviewed did not morally discriminate between different types of *abortions* (earlier versus later term ones, for instance), preferring instead to differentiate between different types of *women* who had abortions and the different kinds of abortion decisions they made. The bottom line is that these women were more than willing to call one another to account morally for what they did and the way they did it—and to judge one another as culpable when certain standards weren't met. What these women understood was that despite its somewhat old-fashioned reputation, morality is as important a concept today as it ever was. Politicians *shouldn't* cut funds to the disabled while quarantining military expenditure. Schools *should* be charged with educating our youth about sex. Ethnic and religious minorities living in the West *should not* be allowed to mutilate the genitals of the young girls in their communities. Every time we say the word "should," we are talking morals, and most of us engage in this sort of talk all the time. We use our moral beliefs to define the kind of people we are, and the kind of world we want to live in. As Julia and Winston—the heroes of George Orwell's *1984*—discovered, acting on our values is as essential to life as food and water, while being unable to act on them cripples our self-respect. For some women, like Lucy, the challenge to her anti-choice views posed by a mature-aged pregnancy and a late period led her to redefine herself as someone tolerant of abortion:

I really went through it a few months back because I thought I was pregnant. It would have been my fourth child, and up until that point I'd been against abortion for myself—I could never imagine I would have one. Many of my mother's friends had to have abortions in the fifties and had gone through hard times. So my mother had a tolerant attitude toward abortion, but I could never imagine myself having one. But then, faced with a three-day-late period, I thought I would have to make a choice.

I'd also had to think about abortion when I had my third child. I was already forty, so I had to have amniocentesis, and it was on my mind that if something was wrong I would have to face that choice. As it turned out, the baby was fine, but it was difficult—I found it was very difficult. But then again, having a fourth child would also have been difficult. Financially, we would have gone down the chute. So now I'm tolerant to abortion. The choice should be there, so you have a say, and are not sent off to the back-yarders. But it's not an easy choice.

On the other hand, it was difficult to miss Carmen's self-hatred —expressed in both words and body language—over what she saw as her inability to act on her anti-choice beliefs:

CARMEN: I know from past experience that I'd have an abortion, even though rationally I'd rather be able to give the baby up for adoption. But in the circumstances you're in a very different state of mind . . . You're very insecure. Vulnerable. Sometimes you just feel that the only way out is to have an abortion. So I know that if I became pregnant, I'd lean towards having an abortion, because that's what I've done before.

LC: Why do you feel it is more rational to give the baby up for adoption?

CARMEN: I prefer the idea of it. I don't think it's morally acceptable to terminate. I don't like the idea of having an abortion. But you were saying, "if that happened to you, what would you do?" That's what I'd end up doing.

A young childcare worker I know was changing a diaper when she learned I was writing a book about women's abortion ethics. "Really!" she said excitedly as she gently tended the bottom before her. "I'd really like to read that!" As I stood before my publisher with my youngest strapped papoose-like to my back, she exclaimed, "We're always talking about babies or abortion. It's so strange!"

I don't think it's strange that a young childcare worker is interested in reading about women's views on abortion, nor that most of my conversations this past year (with my publisher and everyone else!) have been about either babies or abortion. The abortion issue is not separate from the complex web of women's experiences, understandings, and feelings about mothering children, but part of it. Women's decisions about abortion are the same sorts of decisions they make about mothering, only with different outcomes.

I know this not just from researching this book, but from my own experience. When you write about abortion, one of the first questions people ask you is whether or not you've ever had one. I never have, but I have had an unplanned pregnancy. Although in the end my partner and I chose to become parents, there were weeks of uncertainty while we considered, together and separately, whether or not we would be able to be "good enough" parents to our could-be child. Reasons for continuing the pregnancy: we loved each other; we did ultimately want children together. Reasons against: we'd only been together for a year; we had little money; my partner had already booked and paid for an overseas trip of unspecified length. For: we would have the emotional support of his and my parents. Against: we would have little material support from any of them because mine lived overseas and his lived in the country and outer suburbs. For: . . . and so it went on, a decision-making *process* indistinguishable from those gone through by others considering parenthood, and indistinguishable from those gone through by those who ultimately decide in favor of abortion—bar the *decision* that eventually dropped out at the end.

Once I began telling people that I had decided to become a mother, no one ever suggested that this decision had not been mine to make. Nor did I ever question it myself. Perhaps it is our society's overwhelming acceptance of women's decisions *to* mother that makes the distrust many people have of their decisions *not to* so odd. To say that women should decide whether or not they will become mothers is not to say that they aren't responsible for making this decision thoughtfully, carefully, and ethically. Rather, it is to ask who is in a better position to make decisions about motherhood and abortion than the pregnant woman herself?[7]

Women and men are slowly realizing that their fertility—despite the claims of modern medicine—is not easily controllable. Even if modern contraceptive methods were really as simple and liberating to use and as fool-proof as the experts would have us believe, our limited capacity as humans to always act as we should—especially in the sexual arena—will forever stand in the way of completely eliminating unplanned pregnancies. The need for abortion, then, is a need that may fluctuate but will never go away.

What does need to go away, however, are the constant attempts by anti-choice activists and politicians to chip away—or undermine completely—the legal structures that enable women's access to safe abortion services. Women desperately need the abortion issue laid to rest—or at least laid low—so they can pursue other political goals. Naomi Wolf recently argued that the pro-choice movement has lost a sizeable chunk of supporters over the years because it refuses to see abortion as a moral issue. It seems to me that what so many potential pro-choice supporters want to hear—in the slogans and the analysis of the pro-choice movement—is a distinctly moral understanding of what abortion is and when it is, and is not, justified. I agree with Wolf that only when the pro-choice movement expands on its understanding of the meaning and importance of abortion to women will the "middle ground" refuse their support to the forces that seek to demonize abortion and make it illegal, thereby putting the health and safety of women who need them at risk.

The ethic spelled out in this book comes from women in this middle ground, those who know that women must have the right to choose, but recognize that with rights come responsibilities. And it is for women and men on this same turf (recently referred to by a pro-choice personality as the "mushy middle") that I have written it.

# A Note to the Reader

Discussion of abortion has evolved to the point where the use of the terms "pro-life" or "pro-choice" indicates sympathy for one or the other side of the argument. Most researchers and writers in the area recognize they are in a minefield and have thought that the best way out of it is to call each side by its preferred name. I have not chosen this route, however, for the simple reason that I find the term "pro-life" so offensive that I cannot use it without feeling angry: offensive because of its purposeful and highly inaccurate suggestion that those on the opposite side of the argument are enthusiastic supporters of—or "pro"—death. Throughout this book I use the terms "pro-choice" and "anti-choice," which I think give a fairer description of each side's position: either in favor of or opposed to women having the freedom to choose abortion. Readers are warned, however, that some people quoted in the book have made different choices.

## Acknowledgments

I am extremely grateful to the following people for helping me get this book into print. Some helped me with editing and design, some took the time to argue some points, while others supported me in my struggle to forsake academic-speak and write in a more "user-friendly" fashion. In no particular order they are: Jane Usher, Yoni Prior, Tor Roxburgh, Lyn Gillam, Gaby Naher, Sophie Cunningham, Vicki Clarke, Sandy Webster, and Adam Clarke.

This book began life as a Master's thesis, and I have found the comments of the two academics who marked it—Justin Oakley and Catriona Mackenzie—extremely valuable.

I also want to give a special thanks to my father and my partner. This book could never have been written without their generous emotional and financial support.

# Introduction

*The Abortion Myth* was not written as an academic book. It was first published in Australia as a general audience—or "trade"—paperback. I say this at the outset because, while it is extensively researched and I believe touches with adequate complexity on all of the relevant issues and arguments about abortion, the main body of *The Abortion Myth* omits or resists engagement in the intense and often fractious debates around methodology, epistemology, and post-modern discourses about the body, to name a few.

These omissions are not evidence of my disinterest in these subject areas, nor of a view that they are irrelevant to the lay reader. Rather, they reflect my belief that abortion is not primarily an academic subject area, but a real-life medical, moral, and cultural issue that touches the lives of almost every woman, either directly or indirectly. To use real women's experience about abortion to construct a real-world abortion ethic, and then to write a book full of the jargon that functions efficiently as shorthand for academics but sounds like so much gobbledygook to the uninitiated, seemed to me to be an act of paternalistic insensitivity.

Having said all that, the publication of *The Abortion Myth* as an academic book in the United States provides me with a limited opportunity to address some of the academic concerns and issues that were left to one side in the original Australian publication. Thus, in this Introduction I situate *The Abortion Myth* in the context of American scholarship and articulate my understanding of the meaning and value of women's experience to psychological and ethical investigations of the morality of abortion. An appendix can be found in the back of the book for readers interested in more detail about the methodology of the study than is found in the main text. Those not interested in covering any of this ground may wish to skip to the next section, entitled "American Abortion Politics: New Battles in the Same Old War."

## Situating *The Abortion Myth* in the Context of American Scholarship

Where does the scholarship in *The Abortion Myth* fit with all that has come before? Professor Jill Morawski breaks down abortion research into four categories: legal/activist work, philosophies of rights, cultural studies, and psychological investigations of women's experiences.[1] She defines the latter category as sociological and psychological investigations into women's decision making and experience, which are either demographic or designed to investigate the psychological sequelae of women's abortion decisions. She groups *The Abortion Myth* in the same category as studies like Kristin Luker's *Abortion and the Politics of Motherhood*, Fay Ginsburg's *Contested Lives* and Carol Gilligan's *In a Different Voice*—much needed "exceptions" to the thrust of most social scientific work in the area.

I mostly agree with Morawski's categorization of *The Abortion Myth*. Certainly Luker's, Ginsburg's, and Gilligan's work strongly influenced my data collection methods, as well as the way I analyzed the data. But I am also indebted to the scholarship of historian and political scientist Rosalind Petchesky and journalist Janet Hadley, as well as to the work of the Condit sisters, who often employ a cultural studies perspective in their analyses.[2] In fact, I think what Luker and Ginsburg are doing, in many ways, is putting the cultural studies agenda into practice insofar as that agenda may be characterized as the revelation of the historical contingency[3] of culturally crafted[4] social discourses that drive social conflicts like abortion.

In addition to replicating in Australia both Luker's and Ginsburg's conclusions about the concerns that focus the energies of activists involved in the debate—women's changing role in society—my findings suggest that this focus can be found in samples of non-activist as well as activist women (although the self-selectivity of participants in my study makes it likely that the women whose voices form the core of *The Abortion Myth* have a higher than usual level of interest in and concern about abortion).

Yet, while *The Abortion Myth* wholeheartedly supports Luker's and Ginsburg's contention that motherhood is the central issue at play in the abortion debate, it disputes Luker's conclusion that women on both sides of the issue have different views of motherhood and that these differences are the basis for the longevity and bitterness of the debate.[5] Instead, my data suggests that women's understanding and valuing of motherhood is stunningly similar (and some feminists might complain, frustratingly reactionary). Where women critically differ is in their judgments of the moral soundness of "other" women's attitudes, emotionality, and reasons for deciding to abort. For anti-choice women, the paradigmatic aborting women is a youngish, childless "career" woman who has an abortion so her pregnancy won't disrupt a planned ski holiday (read: a woman too selfish, too engaged in a man's world and "male" values, and with too much time and money on her hands). Pro-choice women, on the other hand, were more likely to see women who have abortions as every woman and any woman, and to express reservations about their capacity to judge the moral acceptability of another woman's choice—although they did suggest that the aborting woman herself ought to ensure that her decision met basic community moral standards. And while it should come as no surprise that the above stereotype of the thoughtless and immoral aborting woman is carefully concocted and deliberately disseminated by the anti-choice movement, it is disturbing to realize that some of the pro-choice movement's own explanations and justifications of a woman right to choose inadvertently support this politically debilitating and empirically false stereotype. One of the more hopeful predictions made in *The Abortion Myth* is that the pro-choice movement's successful promotion of an accurate and morally infused vision of women who have abortions will bring to the foreground the view of mothering shared by pro- and anti-choice women. This shared view might then form the basis of a new dialogue on abortion and foster a greater degree of tolerance and coexistence between women than has been seen so far.

## Valuing Women's Experience

Women's views and beliefs about unplanned pregnancies, abortion, and the advent of the artificial womb form the basis of the moral theory articulated in *The Abortion Myth*. It is notable that neither Luker nor Ginsburg feels compelled to provide extensive justification or any justification at all of their use of social actors' narratives—and the interpretations those actors provide of their narratives—to expand current understandings of the nature and meaning of the abortion debate. In the American academy (unlike the academy in Australia), it seems that it is no longer necessary to explain and justify research that gives preference to the interpretations and meanings people give to their own beliefs and behavior over the interpretations imputed to research "subjects" by "objective" researchers. When Ginsburg implores her readers to "Suspend for a moment whatever they have always believed to be the 'truth' in order to listen to voices other than their own," she assumes her audience shares her beliefs about what such a willingness to "enter into the viewpoint" of those "at the coalface" might accomplish.[6] I share Ginsburg's assumptions about the raft of benefits that can accrue to those in direct conflict—and to the larger community— when disputants agree in good faith to empathetically "enter into to the viewpoint" of "the other" side. These include the clearing up of any misunderstandings about the real points at issue in the debate and a sharp decline in the distrust and animosity between those on each side: feelings that both sap the desire for agreement and provide practical obstacles to achieving it.

What Luker and Ginsburg do not claim is that their data provides insights into the morality or otherwise of abortion. It is mainly ethicists, not social scientists, who are interested in answering the question, "Is it moral?" Orthodox ethicists have long assumed that the road to "the right" is through abstracted, logical reflection, reflection that not only ignores the views of those who experience a particular moral dilemma, but attempts to distance itself from the "biased" experience and emotions of the moral expert herself. What this has meant in practice is that the countless ethical forays into abortion largely begin and end with a particular philosopher's "reflection" on the topic, and/or her reflection on the previous reflections of other philosophers. The outcome of this approach is predictable: reams of ethical discourse that seeks to mould the abortion "problem" into one recognizable—and so resolvable—by traditional normative theories and approaches. This approach has led many ethicists to conclude that the conflict around abortion will be resolved once it is ascertained how the philosophically agreed upon moral principle that "it is wrong to kill another person" can be applied to the fetus.[7]

It is orthodox philosophy's indifference to the moral experience of individuals or groups who must actually face particular moral dilemmas in the course of living their lives that lies at the heart of the abstract reflective approach. It is an indifference summed up by the response of a prominent ethicist to my study. When I pointed out to him how women's views and experiences repeatedly contradicted established moral thought on abortion he replied: "Well, who cares what women think? That they think it doesn't make it right."

I fought through the disdain for my research encapsulated by this remark for a number of reasons. First, because I recognized that the systematic use of the life experience and understandings of different groups of people posed fundamental challenges to time-honored philosophical approaches to knowledge generation, and so to time-honored philosophical knowledge. If experience is seen as the basis for philosophical inquiry, the very nature of the questions being asked, as well as the answers being provided, will change. Approaching women in an open-ended manner to inquire about the moral issues surrounding abortion might immediately, for example, place the notion of unexpected pregnancies rather than the act of abortion at the center of the inquiry. Listening to how women evaluate the morality of the range of issues surrounding unexpected pregnancies pushes their attitudes, emotionality, and reasons—rather than the rightness or wrongness of the disembodied act of aborting—to the center of the moral frame.

I also recognized that, however isolated I was in my department, I was not really working alone. I was and continue to be nourished by the work of other feminists, working inside and beyond Australia's borders. For example, while it is true that I disagree with the central (often implied) claim in Gilligan's *In a Different Voice* (that the alternative voice evidenced in women's moral discourse is necessarily female[8]) I recognized that the emphasis women in my study placed on their responsibilities in the abortion decision replicated Gilligan's findings over a decade earlier. Along with this recognition went the more vital awareness that the divergence of women in my study from the familiar rights framework that is the norm in the abortion debate more likely indicated the limitation of that norm than the limitations of women's moral perspective.

I also drew strength from feminist ethicists who have long insisted that what women believe and value offers profound insights into the moral. Standpoint theorists have argued since the 1980s that women's marginalized position in society gives them privileged access to the "truth," although these theories have fallen into disrepute and disuse in the 1990s.[9] Hekman rightly points out that the rise of post-modernism is partially to blame for the decline of Standpoint and argues persuasively that feminists must abandon the quest to establish that women have a corner on the "truth." But as Hekman also notes, while women are no more able than any other group to step outside themselves and see how it "really is," their "partial and perverse" perspective may provide a "definition of a less repressive society" insofar—I would add—as gender is concerned anyway.[10]

Ethicists like Virginia Held and Paul Lauritzen have also dedicated themselves to finding a place for women's experience in moral theory, though both are palpably limited by their assumption that existing normative theories must accommodate lived experience, rather than committing to experience as the starting point for new normative theories.[11] Moreover, neither Held nor Lauritzen—nor any feminist philosopher that I've come across—directly addresses the question of how academics ought to go about finding out how women describe and understand the moral. I believe this issue must be addressed, or women will continue to be spoken for by individuals or small coteries of (usually) female ethicists who, however well-meaning, have no particular claim to knowing what anyone other than themselves believes to be ethical or "true." I believe *The*

*Abortion Myth* offers an example of using women's experience—gathered using the traditional psychological interview method—as the starting point for ethical (and political) reflection. In my view, the goal should be to couple qualitative methods of collecting and arriving at an in-depth understanding of women's experience with quantitative ones to establish the breadth of the moral trends identified amongst different groups of women. Harnessing the strengths of each research method will best enable ethicists to define and understand areas of difference between women of different nationalities, races, social and economic status, and so on. It therefore goes without saying that *The Abortion Myth* is only the first step in what ultimately should be a wider investigation into the prevalence in the wider community—and in the sub-groups within it—of the views expressed by the women I interviewed.

The upshot of all this is that while I believe women may have a privileged perspective on issues surrounding unplanned pregnancy, their privilege doesn't make them objective knowers of universal truths. Instead, I believe that using the knowledge to which this particular contingent of Australian women may have privileged access is how best to maximize the capacity of similar Australian women to fulfil the moral and social responsibilities that surround unplanned pregnancies. We ought to value women's moral framework and moral values around abortion because they are liberatory and useful in resolving real-life moral strife, not because they—or anything for that matter—can claim to be objectively right.

## American Abortion Politics:
## New Battles in the Same Old War

Anyone who has even half an ear tuned to the American political abortion scene has heard about "partial birth" or Dilitation and eXtraction (D&X) second trimester abortions. The rise of this issue to prominence displays the public's—and the politicians'—distrust of women's capacity to think and act morally. It also demonstrates the political and media savvy of the anti-choice movement in once again finding an issue—or more precisely an image and the accompanying rhetoric—that graphically sums up their explicit and implied contentions about women's immorality and their misuse of the freedom to choose abortion. Sadly, the conflict over the D&X procedure also serves as an example of how the pro-choice movement's use of outdated defenses of women's abortion freedoms and its failure to engage with the moral agenda of the anti-choice movement have left it and the women it represents the losers in the social, ethical, and public relations abortion wars.

On the surface, the anti-choice argument against the D&X is simple. Anti-choicers question the "brutal" and "callous" nature of the procedure, which they describe as follows: The doctor turns the "unborn" child into the "breech" position (feet first) and pulls the "child" from the mother until all but the head is delivered. He or she then forces scissors into the base of the skull and inserts a catheter to suction out "the child's" brain.[12]

Such descriptions are standardly accompanied by drawings in which a baby-sized fetus can be viewed—courtesy of the removal of the woman's leg on the viewing side—hanging from a woman's vagina. The pro-choice counter usually entails the assertion that the term "partial-birth abortion" has no medical meaning[13] and an accusation that such anti-choice tactics are inappropriately "ghoulish," "ghastly," and "graphic." It is usually accompanied by warnings that the wording of most "partial birth abortion" legislation will outlaw around 85 percent of all abortion procedures and will critically undermine _Roe v. Wade_'s assertion of a woman's right to choose.[14]

In many ways, the partial-birth campaign is simply a re-run of the tactical approach used so successfully by the anti-choice movement in _The Silent Scream_ and by the fetal-flashing campaigns of the 1980s and early 1990s. The strategy involves making self-conscious assumptions about the self-evident immorality of aborting fetuses that are so "baby-like" in their appearance. It is also a re-run of what I argue in chapters 2 and 3 concerning the largely ineffectual response of the pro-choice movement to these tactics. The "partial-birth" campaign, however, throws a more direct spotlight than has been done previously on the moral complicity and culpability of the aborting woman. "It's bad enough she's having an abortion, and aborting such a baby-like fetus," it is suggested, "but what kind of self-centered and callous woman would choose this sort of procedure to achieve her ends?" Such assertions about women's diminished moral capacities run alongside of—and reinforce—the long-standing anti-choice contention that women have abortions for "convenience." The recent debate in Western Australia on decriminalization of abortion saw one member of Parliament claim that women had abortions because they were "worried about how they would look in their bikinis." Taken together, these arguments suggest that while choice may be a good thing left in the right hands, in the hands of silly, trivial women, choice begets murder. This message was clearly communicated to an anti-choice rally recently when the leader of the Australian anti-choice movement wondered aloud why women having second trimester abortions don't just "go on and allow their baby to be born? I'm sure the Mafia would be happy to kill it for a much cheaper rate."[15]

## Hard Cases Make Bad Law and Impoverished Moral Perspectives

The anti-choice movement has relentlessly and aggressively pushed partial-birth bans, but the pro-choice movement is hopeful that the courts will continue to support challenges to these measures. And while it is critical that the pro-choice movement continue to fight the battle against this most recent anti-choice scourge, it is also imperative that the legal language and concepts used to win this battle be contained within the legal sphere. Thus, while pro-choice lawyers may be compelled to use accepted legal notions like "rights," "privacy," "autonomy," and "choice," and to deny the legal personhood and thus legal relevance of the fetus, the pro-choice movement must recognize the unsuitability of these notions (and the language used to articulate them) in other social arenas where abortion is contested. And this is because, often and perhaps inevitably, the cases that make it to court are those in which a woman has stretched her freedom to the limit, doing things that are as difficult to describe as "choices" as they are to characterize as "responsible" or "ethical."

Cases like the one in Canada in which a woman pregnant with her fourth child refused to enter a drug treatment program, despite the fact that two of her three children had been born with chemical dependence and related developmental problems. Cases like the one in which a woman arrived at the hospital drunk, belligerent, and threatening to kill herself in order to end her near-term pregnancy. Her child, when born, had an elevated blood alcohol level. Or cases like that in which a pregnant woman ignored medical warnings that her drug use would endanger her fetus, only to give birth to a brain-damaged baby who dies soon after. In all these cases, the pro-choice movement has mounted legal arguments that seek to absolve the women involved of legal responsibility for the potential or actual heath problems suffered by their fetuses or children on the grounds that their conduct was "directed at a fetus, not a human being."[16]

Now, I want to make it crystal clear that I am in no way suggesting that women are nothing but "fetal containers" who ought to be jailed for "crimes" against their fetuses. I don't believe that the doctor always knows best, or that society should not be charged with the lion's share of responsibility for the poverty, lack of education, and racism that have contributed to these women's circumstances. Nor am I not suggesting that pro-choice lawyers ought to stop defending any and every woman who risks jail if convicted of "fetal abuse."

But what I *am* saying is that the pro-choice movement needs to leave in the courtroom the defenses and lines of reasoning used to keep pregnant or post-partum women out of jail—defenses that by necessity imply no meaningful relationship, and so no relational responsibility, between the pregnant woman and her fetus. Legal arguments stating that a pregnant woman's behavior is of no consequence because the damaged fetus is or was of no consequence, or because she had a right to do as she wished with her body, or because no one had a right to stop her, have no place outside of an environment in which the only possible roles are that of accuser and accused.

The point is that hard cases make bad law, and they also make bad cases on which to base the pro-choice movement's defense of women's reproductive freedoms. This is because what works to secure women's freedom in the courtroom works to undermine women's moral agency outside of it. The failure of the pro-choice movement to situate women's abortion rights in the context of women's experience and understanding of pregnancy, motherhood, and womanhood has led to a profound alienation of many women from the movement—an alienation that exists despite most women's unwavering belief in their right to choose abortion.

Instead, women's social experience of pregnancy and motherhood, and their moral understanding of that experience, should lie at the heart of pro-choice explanations and justifications for the whole gamut of women's reproductive freedoms in a social, moral, and political context. To this end, I hope *The Abortion Myth* will be useful as a starting point for the creation of concepts and language necessary to articulate a framework that differs radically from—yet is capable of co-existing with—the legal one already in place.

## Clarifications and Updates Since the Australian Publication of *The Abortion Myth*

One misunderstanding that arose from the Australian publication of *The Abortion Myth* was about the required attributes of a moral decision. A friend of mine who works as a clinical psychologist at one of the most reputable abortion clinics in Melbourne rang me after she'd read the book to tell me how much she liked it. "But I'm not sure I agree that all women make moral decisions," she said. "Many of the women I speak to certainly know their own minds." Puzzled, I asked her why abortion decisions made by women who know their own minds aren't moral. "Because moral decisions are uncertain, aren't they? Some of the women I counsel don't hesitate at all when making their decision. And once their minds are made up, that's it."

A moral decision can be made in an instant. A woman can make a moral decision without a shadow of a doubt. For instance, many women who use birth control are clear about their lack of readiness to assume the responsibilities of motherhood: hence the birth control. Should the birth control fail and they become pregnant, this knowledge—and thus their realization that they will choose abortion

—may be instantaneous and unambiguous. In this sort of situation, a clear and quickly made decision is not likely to indicate an immoral choice, but rather one in which the care and thought that characterizes moral choice came earlier, probably when the decision to contracept was made. Other markers of moral decisions—sadness over the need to make the decision at all, and acknowledgment of the seriousness of pregnancy, motherhood, and abortion—may or may not be noticeable to others. But this doesn't matter. While it is important that women as a group—through representative organizations like the pro-choice movement—articulate their belief that abortion is a moral issue, not every woman is required to display to everyone external evidence that she is making a moral decision. What matters is that the woman herself knows that her decision met the standards for moral choice articulated by the community of which she feels herself to be a member.

## An Artificial Womb: You're Dreaming!

Most critics of *The Abortion Myth* viewed the ethical scenario at its center—the invention of an artificial womb for very young fetuses—as little more than an ingenious thought experiment. They dismissed, to a large extent, the possibility of such a contraption coming into being any time in the near future, and so underestimated the urgency attached to my call for the pro-choice movement to disentangle its defense of women's reproductive freedoms from a woman's right to "control her body."[17]

I believe I provide adequate argument in the text that the rapid decline in the number of weeks at which a fetus is considered viable means that many of the horrors that I have predicted will attend development of an artificial womb capable of gestating very young fetuses are already here. However, I would like to bring to the attention of the skeptics several developments suggesting that scientists are managing to find funds to pursue the varied knowledges that will be required to develop a womb that will either gestate very young fetuses taken from their mothers' bodies or will continue the gestation of "test-tube" embryos.

Item: ***Artificial Placenta Work to Begin.*** The National Institute of General Medical Sciences in Washington D.C., part of the National Institute of Health, has given away some part of two million dollars to Ohio State University's Douglas Kniss. Kniss wants to build an artificial placenta by growing cultures of placenta cells in three dimensions on a fabric structure bathed in a blood-like growth medium.[18]

Item: ***Womb Donors Program Needed.*** British surgeons will soon be able to give infertile women a new womb. The surgeons plan to recycle wombs removed from women who have completed their families and implant them in women whose wombs are infertile. Initially, the donor program will only be open to women with congenital abnormalities, or who have undergone cancer treatment.[19]

We can view these developments as evidence of a rapidly closing window of opportunity for change in the way pro-choice feminists defend women's reproductive freedoms, or we can take them as a timely reminder that, where there's a will, there's a way. I think they are both.

*March 1999*

# The Abortion Myth

# · 1 ·

# Is It Right?

The kernel of this book was formed sixteen years ago in the country of my birth, the United States. I had eagerly accompanied my mother to the office of a local senate candidate to stuff envelopes for his re-election push. I don't know if either of us even knew the candidate's name, or what he stood for, beyond the fact that he was pro-choice. This was 1979, and the intentions of a former actor named Ronald Reagan were already written on the wall, though few would have predicted how successful the anti-choice movement would become. If you'd asked me why I cared so passionately about the abortion issue, I almost certainly would have shrugged my fourteen-year-old shoulders in an irritated way and said, "I don't *knooow*."

It's taken me a few years, but I suspect I now do know why the topic of abortion fascinates me. I think when I was younger I knew on some instinctive level what I now know intellectually: that without full reproductive rights—and that includes abortion—women's crusade for freedom and equality is beaten before it's begun. As Susan Faludi put it recently in *Backlash:* "All of women's aspirations —whether for education, work or any form of self-determination— ultimately rest on their ability to decide whether and when to bear children."[1]

But the other reason I was and remain so spellbound by the abortion issue is that I never felt the whole story was being told. Yes, I surely believed—as I do now—that women have a right to choose abortion, but was that really the end of the story? While I felt committed—and had committed myself—over the years to fight for a woman's right to choose, I was unsure if abortion was a choice *I* could ever make. I wanted the right to have an abortion if I needed it, but I didn't ever want to need one.

I remember during high school experiencing a great deal of confusion about these feelings and keeping them to myself for fear that voicing them would lead to my being mistaken for a "right-to-lifer." Later, when I was eighteen and part of the reproductive-rights group of the Manhattan chapter of the National Organization for Women (NOW), I began to search through the NOW bookcases for something that might help me understand the abortion issue and my own feelings about it a bit better. Little I found was of any help. The woman's movement was firmly behind a woman's right to "control her body" by choosing abortion, and if anyone felt anything less than total comfort with the explanation and defense of this position, they weren't talking. Nobody said it, but I got the feeling that to deviate from the stated position of the movement was to give comfort to the enemy—the far, anti-feminist right. This was 1983, and the power and influence of the enemy was fast on the rise. It seemed better, for the moment, to shut my mouth.

So I did, and argued the standard pro-choice position in a variety of campus forums, both as a NOW member, and later, as a student at Wesleyan University. But probably because my questions about the ethics of abortion had still not been articulated, much less answered, my fascination with the issue remained. In 1989, several years after I graduated from university, I emigrated to Australia and enrolled in a Master's degree at the Centre for Human Bioethics at Monash University in Melbourne. The final requirement of the degree was the production of a 10,000-word thesis. As I recall, I didn't find the topic for the thesis, it found me.

## The Ectogenetic "Solution"

I found my thesis topic while reading a text by Professor Peter Singer, a prominent ethicist who was the director of the Centre at the time. In *The Reproduction Revolution*, Singer and his co-author, Deane Wells, speculated that the gestation of very young fetuses in artificial wombs (a process they called ectogenesis) would resolve the conflict surrounding abortion. By an ectogenetic womb, the authors were referring to an artificial womb, much like the humidicribs or incubators currently in use in neo-natal wards. Singer and Wells wrote that, in the near future, technological advances would mean that younger and younger "premmies" would become "viable," able to be kept alive outside their mothers' wombs. Twenty years ago, babies who'd spent less than twenty-eight weeks in the maternal womb had little chance of surviving (a usual pregnancy lasts forty weeks), but today neonatologists are proudly "rescuing" babies as young as twenty-two weeks.[2]

Singer and Wells point out that since the anti-choice movement objects to abortion because it kills the fetus, an incubator capable of saving the lives of very young fetuses would likely meet with their approval: "Ectogenesis could at some future time make right-to-life organizations drop their objections to abortion; for it is only our inability to keep early foetuses alive that makes abortion synonymous with the violation of any right to life that the foetus may have."[3]

According to the authors, the women's movement would also be compelled to welcome ectogenetic technology. A woman's right to control her body is the basis of feminist arguments for abortion rights, and the artificial womb would enable women to have that control, without forcing them to terminate the lives of their fetuses. A woman's right to choose an abortion, the authors implied, was simply and only a right to decide whether or not her *pregnancy* should continue. It was not the right to decide whether her *fetus* would live and, therefore, whether or not she would become a *mother*. The authors said that when the ectogenetic womb made it possible to end an early pregnancy without killing the fetus, it would be unethical for a woman to make the latter choice. A woman faced with an unwanted pregnancy, in other words, should only be given the choice to *evacuate* the fetus to an artificial womb, adopt the child out when it was born, or take on the responsibilities of motherhood. Singer and Wells said that traditional abortion—and the death of the fetus it entails—would no longer be an ethical option for women because "freedom to choose what is to happen to one's body is one thing; freedom to insist on the death of a being that is capable of living outside one's body is another." The artificial womb, the authors believed, would end the abortion conflict as we know it, leaving "pro-choice feminist and pro-foetus right-to-lifers [to] . . . embrace in happy harmony."[4]

It is important to realize that the implications of ectogenesis go well beyond potential group hugging sessions between pro- and anti-choice activists. If babies are no longer fully gestated in the bodies of their mothers, then it no longer makes sense to claim—as feminists do—that abortion is solely a woman's right because it takes place solely in a woman's body. While women could still argue that their ownership of their bodies gave them the right to decide whether or not they would choose ectogenesis in the first place, once their fetus was in the artificial womb, any number of "interested parties"—genetic fathers, doctors, grandmothers-to-be—could also claim "rights" to it. One nightmare scenario (among many) that could result from this redefinition of women's abortion rights is that a pregnant woman, denied the right to choose abortion (where the fetus dies), chooses to evacuate her fetus to an ectogenetic womb in preference to bringing the pregnancy to term. When the tiny fetus is born, the doctor who examines it concludes that it is severely damaged and is likely to either die a long painful death or live a severely disabled life. While the woman wants to shut down her fetus's ectogenetic life-support (allowing the fetus to die), her estranged husband (the genetic father) argues strenuously for keeping the fetus hooked up. Court proceedings follow and . . . you get the picture, I'm sure.

Of course, some would argue that the equalizing of men's and women's relationships with their fetuses is an *advantage* ectogenesis has over pregnancy. It seems to me, however, that this argument only works if it is clear that men have the right motives for wanting to have such close involvement with decisions about their could-be children. Sadly, current research suggests that it is precisely the men who are likely to seek such close involvement whose motives are most questionable. Researchers in separate studies done in the Netherlands, Australia, Canada, and the United States, for example, have found that men who joined "fathers' rights movements" were "angry men: angry about paying out what they consider to be huge sums of money in child support, angry that they have limited access to their children, and angry with the whole divorce and child custody process. They join fathers' rights groups for personal reasons and for personal gain."[5] Under the guise of seeking greater involvement in and responsibility for their children's lives, fathers' rights activists tie up the courts in attempts to re-assert control over their kids and their ex-wives. One man, for example, explains why he's a fathers' rights activist this way: "I mean, I hate to see my relationship with my child defined in terms of power. But my ex has all the power. She has all the marbles and I'm constantly kowtowing. And I don't like it."[6] A similar sense of victimization also characterizes this activist:

Can I say anything about my wife to my children? No. She did a bad thing. She committed rape of a father and the love between him and his children. That is what she did . . . It was not only a rape of my children; it is also a rape of my resources. I was the one that went through university. I worked hard for where I am right now. She didn't. She got her job and she is working, but it is not as much as I am getting.[7]

The conclusion of the Canadian study differs little from that drawn by other researchers doing similar studies. It is a warning to all those expecting things to be warm and fuzzy between genetic fathers and pregnant women in the post-ectogenesis era:

Fathers' rightists are not lobbying for joint, equal responsibility and care of children . . . Fathers' rightists have coopted the language of equality but not the spirit of equality. [In] their own words, fathers [told] us that they do not want sole responsibility for children, nor do they want an equal division of child care and responsibility . . . Indeed, fathers want to play a role in their children's lives; but for most, that role is . . . [one] of the traditional father who exercises his power and control.[8]

## Of Abortions and Violins
### (or, Philosophers Say the Weirdest Things)

Did Singer and Wells really think the artificial womb would end the abortion conflict? I must admit, even after all these years, I still find this conclusion astounding. Back then, I was nearly paralytic with confusion and outrage. These two feelings would, in fact, be my constant companions as I painfully sought to change from a social-science perspective—I was a psychology major at Wesleyan—to a philosophical one. It wasn't easy. The social sciences teach you that what is interesting to know about is what people actually *do* in the world, and how their behavior can be predicted by where they come from, what they've learned, or what they say they believe. To find out what people do requires that you ask them about, or, preferably, monitor their behavior. Nearly everything a social scientist thinks is worth knowing is learned from studying people's behavior.

A philosopher, on the other hand, is a beast of an entirely different nature. What she thinks is worth knowing is that which is arrived at after careful and highly abstract reflection. Human behavior is not observed, but rather assumed, so that it may be dissected into its constituent parts for further analysis and judgment. Ethical judgments are typically arrived at as a result of logical steps from an initial "premise," which is either deemed to be self-evident or is presented as a "given" that must be accepted for the sake of further argument. All this abstraction means that philosophers often tend to lose sight of the people at the heart of moral issues. Says Kathleen McDonnell, a feminist concerned with the ethics of abortion: "To read some of the moral theory on abortion . . . is to be uncomfortably reminded of the old caricature of the Catholic theologians debating bow many angels could dance on the head of a pin. One wants to cry out that there is a real woman involved here, facing a real dilemma, experiencing real anguish."[9]

In most ethical argument, appeals to personal experience ("a woman I knew . . ."), highly selective examples, and contrived analogies are substituted for actual human experience. A good example of argument by analogy can be found in a well-regarded article by feminist ethicist Judith Jarvis Thomson. In "A Defense of Abortion" Thomson "grants" what is usually considered the central point of argument in the abortion debate—that the fetus *is* a person from conception. She then argues that even if the fetus is a person, this does not logically lead (as is usually assumed) to the conclusion that the mother is morally obligated to *support* that right. She makes this argument with an analogy about a violin player:

Imagine . . . you wake up in the morning and find yourself back to back in bed with a [famous] unconscious violinist. He has been found to have a fatal kidney ailment, and the Society of Music Lovers has canvassed all the available medical records and found that you alone have the right blood type to help. They have therefore kidnapped you, and last night the violinist's circulatory system was plugged into yours, so that your kidneys can be used to extract poisons from his blood as well as your own. The director of the hospital tells you "Look, we're sorry the Society of Music Lovers did this to you—we would never have permitted it if we had known. But still, they did it, and the violinist now is plugged into you. To unplug you would be to kill him. But never mind, it's only for nine months. By then he will have recovered from his ailment, and can safely be unplugged from you."[10]

The point of the analogy is to demonstrate that while a woman would be "kind" not to pull the plug on the violinist, she certainly couldn't be faulted if pull the plug she did. The analogy is meant to prove that, even if the fetus has a right to life, morally a woman's body can't be conscripted to support it.

There are two things that must be said about the violin scenario. The first is a warning: resist getting sucked in! It's human nature to struggle, when reading an analogy, to make it work. To see, in other words, the ways in which the situation of the conscript to the violinist's cause is like the situation of the pregnant woman vis-à-vis her fetus. Try reading it again, looking this time not for what works about the analogy, but what doesn't. How would a real woman's experience of pregnancy stack up against the forced bed-rest endured by the conscriptee? How does the analogy account for the sex required to make a pregnancy in the first place? How comparable is the way most women actually feel about pregnancy, their fetuses, and impending motherhood and the way the conscriptee is likely to be feeling about the violinist? Allowing the analogy—which is a mismatch with women's experience of pregnancy in so many important ways—to stand in for data investigating how women actually experience and understand their relationship with the fetus in pregnancy, is to erase women from the abortion debate. Because the whole point of making the analogy is to draw conclusions about the moral acceptability of abortion, the omission of women's experience of pregnancy is (to say the least) extremely worrying.

The second problem with the violinist analogy is that it ultimately forces a feminist like Thomson to agree with Singer and Wells that ectogenesis is a better—read morally superior—solution to unwanted pregnancy than abortion. Thomson herself acknowledges this at the conclusion of her article: "I have argued that you are not morally required to spend nine months in bed, sustaining the life of the violinist; but to say this is by no means to say that if, when you unplug yourself, there is a miracle and he survives, you then have a right to turn around and slit his throat." If the fetus is able to survive outside its mother's body, in other words, a woman's desire for it to die cannot morally, according to Thomson, be "gratified."

Sadly, Thomson is not the only feminist who has found herself sucked into supporting ectogenesis. In her book *Ethics and Human Reproduction: A Feminist Analysis*, ethicist Christine Overall's prior logical commitment to the belief that "the pregnant woman (or anyone else, e.g., a physician) has no right to kill the . . . fetus" leaves her with no other option than to grit her teeth (you can almost hear the grinding in her reluctant prose) and go along with the suggestion that once fetal death is no longer the inevitable outcome of abortion, traditional abortion (where the fetus dies) becomes a moral crime.[11]

## The Study

The problem with Singer and Wells's ectogenetic solution is that it is perfectly logical. *If* you buy into the conflicting rights scenario favored by the academics and activists on both sides, ectogenesis seems the solution to the problem of abortion both sides describe. What I suspected, however, was that pro-choice and anti-choice women wouldn't find that ectogenesis solved the abortion problem for *them* at all. If this were so, it would mean that the ethical problems abortion poses for women—regardless of which side they are on—are not as they have been described by the pro- and anti-choice movements. I was struck by the possibility that the inevitable advance of technology could lead to women losing the capacity to decide if and when they would become mothers, leaving them with only the more limited ability to decide the future of their pregnancies. I suspected that the lowering age of viability was already causing problems for women carrying viable or near-viable fetuses, whether those women were wanting later-term abortions, a say in the way they gave birth, or a painless and dignified death for their pre-term fetus. If this slow but steady encroachment into women's rights and responsibilities was to be halted, the women's movement was going to need to change the way it justified a woman's right to choose—and fast. The movement needed to adopt a justification for abortion choice that championed a woman's right to make decisions not only about whether she would continue her pregnancy but about whether her fetus would live or die. Whether or not, in other words, a woman would become a mother.

I decided to conduct a study to discover what women thought of the ectogenetic "solution." I wanted to ask women if they would choose ectogenesis over the current options—abortion, adoption, or keeping the child—currently available to women with unplanned pregnancies. I wanted to use women's own words to explain their views on abortion. Would women describe the abortion issue in ethical terms? If they did, would they use the ethical language of the pro- and anti-choice movements? Would pro-choice women expound on their rights to control their bodies? Would anti-choice women be primarily concerned with the "rights to life" of fetuses? Or would women describe an alternative abortion ethic, one with important differences from the ones with which we are all too familiar and which are heading toward a collision with technological change.

To find out, I had to do what is done so rarely in abortion research; I had to ask women about their views and experience of abortion, and how they made sense of the issue ethically. One researcher who does use women's experiences as research data is Kristin Luker, an eminent American sociologist and author of two books about abortion.[12] In 1975 she noted that her decision to interview women and use their perceptions as significant data in a study of unplanned pregnancy was a ". . . radical departure from most contraceptive and abortion-oriented research. In large part, research on these women and the delivery of services to them has been carried out by people who have never had an unwanted pregnancy—the majority of them, in fact, are incapable of having an unwanted pregnancy because they are men."[13]

More than twenty years after Luker wrote these words, it remains fair to say that while the gender ratio among abortion researchers has shifted somewhat, researchers' attitudes toward the "usefulness" of women's experiences are depressingly similar. In order to enable women to reveal their experiences and understandings, I needed to provide them with a forum that would enable them to uncover and articulate their abortion ethics. The questions I posed had to be unusual enough to make it difficult for them to provide me with pat answers, and the environment safe enough that women committed to either side of the debate would feel comfortable to say what they thought, even if it violated the position taken by their respective movements.

To his credit, Professor Singer agreed to supervise the study—which essentially sought to discredit his speculation about ectogenesis solving the abortion conflict. I designed a number of imaginary moral dilemmas that would give participants a chance to discuss their views on abortion and the ectogenetic solution. The central question I asked the women was what they would do if they became unexpectedly pregnant and were offered the possibility of ectogenesis in addition to the traditional abortion and adoption options—and why. I also asked women to imagine what they'd do if they were asked to donate fetal tissue, or to abort an intended pregnancy to win a trip overseas to the Olympics. Ultimately, I interviewed forty-five women of childbearing age—approximately half of them were pro-choice and half of them anti-choice.

Women were interviewed in groups, with somewhere between five and ten women attending each session. The women were a diverse lot, with a wide range of religious, educational, social, and economic backgrounds. Some had children, others did not. Some had partners, others were single or divorced. Most were in their twenties or early thirties, though several were nearing the end of their childbearing years. One-third of them had previously had an abortion.[14]

## Doing Abortion Research in the 1990s

Before beginning the interview process, I was required to obtain approval to conduct the study from the university ethics committee. Because it was about abortion, the project was automatically classified as high-risk, and I was required to attend an interview with the full committee. I was startled when the chairman—a distinguished pediatrician and neonatologist—asked me for a copy of the final report. He was interested, he said, because he "never could understand how women could abort their babies."

Comments like this made me well aware of how important it was that women-centered abortion research was conducted, and the results broadcast far and wide. But doing abortion research, I quickly discovered, wasn't easy. There were two reasons for this. The first was that in the late 1980s—when I was working on this project—abortion research was taboo. Although Australia had none of the official restrictions of the United States (where abortion-related research was denied Federal funding during the Reagan years), there remained a sense among funding bodies and ethics committees that such research was too controversial to be supported. In fact, prestigious funding bodies like the Australian Health and Medical Research Council *still* don't fund abortion research. Between 1988 and 1995, not one biomedical or public health abortion research project was funded through the NHMRC, which funds over 25 percent of all health and medical research done in Australia. In 1992, the now disbanded women's committee of the NHMRC insisted on a report concerning abortion (it had been fifty-five years since the Council had last considered the issue). When the report was produced, however, the Council refused to endorse it. Says panel member and one-time abortion provider and activist Jo Wainer: "It is almost unprecedented for the Council to [refuse to endorse a report]. It seems that some members of the Council abandoned their responsibility for public health and instead allowed judgments to be made on the basis of a pre-existing moral stance about the rightness or otherwise of abortion."[15]

Without the Council's endorsement, the women's committee feared the Liberal government would not even consider the thirty recommendations made in the report. Unfortunately, these fears were justified. On 18 May 1997 a spokesman for the health minister, Dr. Michael Wooldridge, confirmed that "the Government would not be considering the recommendations because [the report] was not an endorsed document."[16]

Luckily, my degree was self-funded, so I avoided the hurdle of financing the project through the NHMRC or other official funding channels. I also deliberately recruited women for my study from the general public, rather than from institutions with their own ethical hoops to jump, like hospitals or clinics. By this time, I'd managed to secure approval from the university ethics committee, and I didn't want to push my luck.

The second challenge was to ensure that my research acknowledged and moved on from previous contributions of other researchers in the area. This is a standard requirement for academic studies—if you want a passing grade. In my case, however, this proved difficult because the existing work was done in ways that made it of little use to me. As I mentioned before, the *raison d'être* of social science research is to predict behavior. The dominant belief among sociologists and many psychologists is that it is a person's social characteristics—in contrast to their personality or personal history—that determines their behavior. So when social scientists study abortion they ask women their age, the number of years they spent getting educated, how many children they have, the region of the country they hail from, etc. Often the goal of such research seems not to be an increase in knowledge about women's experiences of abortion, but a search for information that will help lower abortion rates. This means that women are asked to tick boxes in questionnaires that reflect views on abortion held by a particular researcher or academic research community. For example, in a study of race differences in abortion attitudes, the answers women give to such difficult questions as "Do you think it should be possible for a pregnant woman to obtain a legal abortion if there is a strong chance of a serious defect in the baby?" are reduced by the researchers to a code ranging from zero (opposition to abortion) to six (approve abortion). Rigid statistical principles are then applied to cross-tabulate these codes against a woman's age, religion, education, and place of birth. Ultimately, conclusions are drawn such as "black and white childbearing women do not differ significantly in their abortion attitudes although race differences appear among older women and men."[17]

What social scientists studying abortion tend *not* to ask women

—as the above study so vividly demonstrates—are the ways in which they make meaning of their life experiences. This precludes them from asking and then speculating upon the larger issues around abortion, like the ethical understanding women have of abortion. While there's little doubt that the "tick a box" method makes the tabulation of results easier and, arguably, the results more accurate, what is gained in ease and "objectivity" is lost in the capacity of the findings to allow women to talk about something the researchers hadn't thought of. In addition, a fair bit of oversimplification and distortion takes place when complex responses to complicated questions are forcibly reduced to numbers.

The one other study that has explicitly sought to understand women's *ethical* approach to abortion is the "abortion decision study" conducted by Harvard moral psychologist Carol Gilligan and reported in her book *In a Different Voice*. Gilligan's work has been very influential among feminist academics, and rightly so. She pointed out the sexism in everything from psychological research methods (the only subjects being used in research were young, white, college-aged men, but the results were generalized to everyone else), to the way decisions are made about what does and does not count as moral thought. Morality, Gilligan argued, reflected the male obsession with abstract principles like "it's wrong to steal" and "abortion is murder." Female moral reasoning, on the other hand, was more holistic, taking into account all the different moral angles—and the numerous practical repercussions—of one course of action rather than another. Women make decisions with their feet on the ground, in other words, not with their ideals in the air. Gilligan's study showed that women faced with an unwanted pregnancy don't ask "Is abortion right?" (an abstract question about moral principles), but "Would abortion be the right thing for me to do in this situation, given who I am and what my life is like?" Take the abortion decision made by Ann:

My husband and I talked about the possibility that I might be pregnant . . . [and] the possibility of abortion . . . It wasn't easy and I didn't feel comfortable with the idea. It wasn't simply a matter of deciding whether or not to have the baby but making that decision in light of the "whole picture," including the marriage relationship . . . I'm [now] in the process of separating [from my husband] . . . I could have had the baby. We might have stayed married or we might have separated, but either way life would have become complicated and messy. I felt I was in an impossible situation.[18]

Gilligan found that not only do many women reason contextually, they find it *immoral* to do otherwise. They would think it wrong, for example, to condemn a woman for aborting if there was no actual financial or emotional support available for the child once it was born. Gilligan was also one of the first to point out that the central moral value in women's abortion decisions is responsibility, not rights. For women, the ideal moral solution is one in which no one gets hurt. When that is not possible—as is the case in decisions about unplanned pregnancies—the best decision is one that identifies and fulfills a woman's obligations to herself, her family, and to "people in general."[19]

Not only do most studies of abortion lack women's voices, they also seem to assume that if a woman does not want to mother, abortion is her only option. Again, I wanted to know more. I was interested not only in why women felt they could not parent (too poor, too many other children, abusive husband, deteriorating relationship), but why, for almost all, abortion—not adoption—was the preferred option.

In the end, my reading of the abortion literature left me with the distinct impression that while there's been a lot of talking *about* and lecturing *to* women about abortion over the years, there hasn't been a hell of a lot of listening to them. I wanted my study to be different. By providing women with a forum to describe their experiences and how they make sense of them ethically, I sought to give women the chance to shape the abortion issue themselves, using their own ethical parameters and terms. After all, I reasoned, it was their perspective on the abortion issue that I wanted to describe, not my own.

## This Book

This book is built around the answers the women I interviewed gave to my questions. Their answers are important, not only because they offer important insights into the moral lens through which women view the abortion issue, but because they suggest some unique solutions to many of the ethical dilemmas posed by the abortion issue as it is traditionally conceived. The "world view" of abortion sketched by the women in this study will be of particular interest to feminists, who pride themselves on listening to women and gearing political action and strategy to the realities of women's lives.

In some senses, the views of the women expressed in this book may be the voices of a new generation. Is there really a feminist generation gap? A number of feminists certainly seem to think so. In the United States, writers like Rene Denfield and Kate Roiphe have published books that challenge conventional feminist wisdom, while in Australia, Virginia Trioli's *Generation F* and Kathy Bail's *DIY Feminism* are the latest entrants into the generational row provoked by feminist stalwarts like novelist Helen Garner and Anne Summers.

It is not surprising that the different experiences of abortion had by older and younger women have led to different political philosophies and goals. A recent television documentary on the underground abortion service operating in the late 1960s and early 1970s in Chicago, known as "Jane," is an important reminder of how different things were for women just twenty-five years ago. Lorraine, who later became a Jane abortion counselor, remembered the era prior to legalization: "It was really a time when if you needed an abortion for whatever reason you took your life in your hands. And you were terrified. Absolutely terrified. All you knew was that you might die. That this person didn't know what he was doing and you were going to bleed to death in a hotel room."

Sunny Chapman recalled the pain and humiliation women seeking illegal abortions experienced:

I went to a doctor who just treated me like dirt. He said "If you girls would keep your legs together you wouldn't have to come in here until after you're married" . . . Everybody I knew that had become pregnant and didn't want to have a baby and had tried to abort had done something really painful and horrible. And they were all hysterical and desperate. Just like I was. Hysterical and desperate and scared.

The power of these memories for many older women led them to worry that younger women take these hard-won freedoms for granted. In the words of one older pro-choice activist:

I get angry because I know so many young women lawyers and doctors and they are the smuggest bunch of people. And I think, "Oh my God they haven't the faintest idea how people fought so they could get into that kind of law school" . . . It's too easy to reach maturity when [legal abortion] is an accomplished fact, like it's always been there for you. And that is the mentality you are talking about on the abortion issue that this group coming up is going to have. How long has it been? [From] 1969? . . . A lot of people became adults during that time and I guess we have to accept that's the way life is.[20]

Not all older feminists, however, feel this way. British health activist and feminist author Sue O'Sullivan, for instance, believes that it is essential that each generation "re-imagines" its own abortion politics: "I think the 1990s has illustrated the fact that nothing is forever and that it's been a mistake politically to think 'well, we've won the right to choose, it's going to be here forever.' We now know this is not the case. In order to keep hold of our hard won rights, we need new ways of imagining things."[21]

The younger women I interviewed tended to see safe and legal abortion as their birthright and were more concerned with the morality of the abortion decisions made by individual women. I would wager that a real threat to women's freedom to choose abortion would most likely unite women—old and young—around the basic goal of safe and legal abortions once more. But while abortion is largely safe and accessible, the morality of women's abortion decisions will remain the hottest topic in the debate.

When viewed through the eyes of the women in this study, abortion metamorphosed into an issue about which women seem to share similar ethical values and concepts, although the way they prioritize these values differs greatly. No matter what their position on the morality of abortion, the women had almost identical views on the ethical issues that should be central in the mind of a woman dealing with the dilemma of an unexpected pregnancy and the concepts pregnant women needed to use to navigate this dilemma: responsibility, motherhood, relationship, caring.

We are a long way from the world of my dreams, where abortion was a hard-fought fight won long ago, and women have turned their attention to other issues of vital concern to their personal well-being and the well-being of their families (extended, paid, penalty-free maternity leave; greater access to low-cost quality childcare and to high-status, well-paid employment spring immediately to mind). But any hope of shelving the abortion issue (even temporarily, and in however untidy a box) rests on a sincere willingness to first have a good hard look at the full scope of what we hope to pack away. While some aspects of the abortion issue have been discussed and analyzed to death, others have been in the "too hard" basket for way too long. For many pro-choice supporters, the thunder of many of these unanswered questions has simply become too loud to ignore: are there "irresponsible" pregnancies? Which reasons for having an abortion are bad ones? Does the fetus matter, how much, and why? Even if women have a right to choose abortion, is it always right for them to do so?

Why, after all this time, have these questions never been answered, and so rarely been asked?

## · 2 ·

# The Way It Is Now

Before delving into the hotly contested arena of abortion politics, a few basic facts about women's access to abortion and their legal rights may be in order. I'll start with the United States. There, the anti-choice movement has turned its attention to eroding women's access to abortion services by both practical and legislative means, having realized that it was unlikely to see its dream of prohibiting abortion legally (either through the adoption by Congress of the "Human Life" amendment or the overthrowing of the *Roe v. Wade* Supreme Court decision legalizing abortion). The most prominent and most successful tactic of the erosion strategy has been the stalking and harassment of abortion providers, the fire bombing of abortion clinics, and the murder of abortion providers. At last count, the American National Abortion Federation had compiled evidence for the following list of anti-choice crimes against abortion-clinic premises and staff: at least 5 murders, 41 bombings, 94 arson attacks, 68 attempted bombings or arson attacks, 547 clinic invasions, 587 acts of vandalism, 95 assaults, 226 death threats, 2 kidnappings, 34 burglaries, 210 incidents of stalking, 1833 pieces of hate mail sent or phone calls made, and 312 bomb threats. Some abortion providers have been forced to hire security guards to protect them from anti-choice extremists, and most work behind bullet-proof glass. Over fifty doctors refused to appear on a recent "60 Minutes" episode about abortion-clinic violence because of fear of reprisals. In October 1998, Buffalo abortion provider Dr. Barnett Slepian was assassinated by an anti-choice zealot in front of his children.

Not surprisingly, recent statistics show that nearly 50 percent of doctors who used to perform abortions in the United States have simply closed up shop. Many have been unable to afford the high levels of security required to practice safely. Others are simply afraid for their lives and the lives of their families. The "greying" of the remaining providers is also cause for concern, especially given the extremely low rates of abortion training in medical schools (only 15 percent make it a mandatory subject). Rick Hudson, author of a recent report on access to abortion and contraception in Canada (where the problems are similar), says that he "draw[s] no confidence from the professional morality of medicine . . . It's very easy to drive gynecologists out of provision because they can make just as much money doing less controversial things."[1]

Another problem with attracting and keeping abortion providers is that it is both low-status and relatively low-paid work. Perhaps most importantly, it is now only older providers who remember what it felt like to watch young women and girls die from septic backyard abortions. As a consequence, nearly 90 percent of counties in the United States don't have an abortion provider, despite being home to over one-third of women between the ages of fifteen and forty-four.

Polling of the American public suggests a burgeoning middle ground. The 1995 Women's Equality Poll found that 74 percent of those polled support women's abortion rights, with only 18 percent opposing women's right to choose. Interpreting these numbers is difficult (a lot depends on the way the questions are asked), but these figures—while showing that a majority of Americans are in favor of choice—suggest a steep decline in support for women's choice, the first decline after years of steadily increasing support. In 1990, the number of Americans who thought abortion should be legal in any or some circumstances was 84 percent. In 1988 it was only 81 percent, while in 1981 it was just 75 percent. Those who believe abortion should be illegal under any circumstances has dropped from 21 percent in 1981 to 17 percent in 1988, and from 12 percent in 1990 to 9 percent in 1992.

In Australia, the continuing legal ambiguity surrounding abortion has not, on the whole, impeded women's access to a safe—though somewhat pricey—first-trimester abortion service. While three quarters of all abortions in Australia are performed in private clinics, Medicare (the Australian universal health insurance scheme) typically pays only a fraction of the costs of a private abortion. In addition, studies have found that 10 percent of eligible clients don't claim the Medicare rebate, largely because of concerns about their privacy. Until recently, many women in both Tasmania and the Australian Capital Territory have had to travel interstate for services, but the opening of new clinics in both regions is likely to alleviate these problems. A recent study of abortion access across the country found that of all Australian women, those who live in the country have the most trouble getting a safe and affordable abortion. Although a system exists to reimburse country women for the costs of travelling to a city for their abortion, a technical glitch in the referral process means most are ineligible. In addition, women from small towns with only one GP often travel to obtain their abortion referral in order to protect their privacy.[2]

Compared to the tens of thousands of members that extreme anti-choice groups attract in the United States, their Australian equivalents number less than five hundred. As a consequence, interference from anti-choice activists outside clinics is rare, and violence unheard of. Nonetheless, Australian groups have been known to adopt less noticeable but equally desperate and deceptive tactics to stop women having abortions. The main one is to list their "pregnancy help centers" with the abortion clinics in the telephone directory. According to one of their senior counselors, when a woman rings seeking abortion they "talk around the issue" with her, using the "opportunity" to misinform her about the health risks associated with abortion (in reality, statistically far less than those associated with childbirth). What they won't tell her is about the availability of abortion or the location of the closest genuine clinic.[3]

A 1996 AGB McNair poll found that a vast majority of Australians (77 percent) believe that the abortion decision should be left to the individual and her doctor. This support, however, is not unequivocal and may be waning. A 1995 Morgan Gallup poll found that approval of abortion for "unmarried mothers," for "married couples," and of "physically handicapped" fetuses had dropped in the last three years by an average of 5 percent.

In Britain, the National Health Service (NHS) is meant to provide

75 percent of all abortion services, though a Royal Commission into the NHS found that in 1993 only 60 percent of abortions were done in the public system with the rest performed in private clinics. David Nolan, of the U.K. Birth Control Trust, says the biggest problems facing women seeking abortions in Britain are "obstructionism by some anti-choice doctors" and "long waiting lists or a limited amount of time and funds set aside by hospitals for abortions." In addition, Nolan says that it is often "very difficult" for a woman to find a doctor to carry out a mid-trimester abortion anywhere in England or Scotland.[4]

A 1995 survey of British public opinion found that 66 percent believed that current abortion laws needed to be changed to allow women an abortion on request, rather than on the signed permission of two doctors. In another survey, however, a much larger number (90 percent) were in favor of women having the right to choose an abortion in the early months of pregnancy in certain (unspecified) circumstances. This is up from 80 percent in 1988, 74 percent in 1983 and 62 percent in 1973.

## Traditional Arguments For and Against Abortion

In recent years, the abortion debate has become all too familiar, and all too predictable. The anti-choice movement claims the fetus has a right to life, the pro-choice movement that it doesn't, or that a woman's right to control her body overrides any claim made by the fetus. Setting up the argument this way places unanswerable questions about the status of the fetus central to the debate: Is the fetus alive? Is it human? Does it have the same ethical rights as people? When the anti-choice movement was in its infancy, it acknowledged these questions as ones of value—not fact—and provided biblically based answers. When this God-centered approach proved unpopular with the political mainstream, however, they switched tactics. Suddenly, questions about the status of the fetus could be answered by "facts" provided by "science." This trend has been commented upon by noted feminist historian Rosalind Petchesky: "Aware of cultural trends, the current leadership of the anti-abortion movement has made a conscious strategic shift from religious discourses and authorities to medico-technical ones, in its effort to win over the courts, the legislatures and popular 'hearts and minds.'"[5]

Though such a switch in emphasis has been politically expedient, the anti-choice movement was disappointed it didn't hand them the game, set, and match. This is because while it is certainly a fact that the fetus is alive (as is a leaf, a slug, and a virus), and is genetically human (it's got a human genetic code and human parents), what exactly this says about the importance of the fetus (and therefore what should and should not be done with it) remains unclear. Essentially, the fetal-centered framework requires anti-choice supporters to "prove" that the fetus is a *person* to demonstrate that abortion is wrong. If the fetus is a person, then it has a right to life. Abortion is wrong because it kills the fetus, and should be made illegal—once again.

It's worth noticing that the right-to-life case can be made without once mentioning the pregnant woman, the woman who is nurturing the fetus in her body and who will be its mother once it is born. If we weren't so used to it, the side lining of women in the drama of pregnancy and birth, and the obliteration of the relationship between the woman and her fetus and could-be child, would be ludicrous. As it stands, we mostly tend not to notice.

One of the reasons we tend not to notice is that the anti-choice movement has been successful in making its definition of the abortion debate *the* definition of the abortion debate. We have come to share their assumption that rights are the only ethical currency that can be used to discuss abortion, and to accept the anti-choice piece of absurdity that pregnant women are their fetuses' adversaries. We have even come to accept the label "pro-life," despite the rising body count from anti-choice clinic violence and the fact that the vast majority of members of anti-choice groups oppose gun reform and are in favor of the death penalty. The truth is that abortion can be supported or opposed without resorting to rights-talk or zeroing in on the status of the fetus. Every time pro-choice supporters accept these terms and argue for abortion choice from within this framework, they concede an important victory to the foes of women's reproductive freedom.

## Morality and the Law

The abortion debate is dominated by rights-talk in large part because of the influence of American feminists on abortion debates in other Western nations. The American obsession with rights is well known and is especially prominent in discussions about abortion because the United States judicial decision that gives women the right to choose is founded on the right to privacy implied in the Constitution. The 1973 Supreme Court decision in *Roe v. Wade* technically left the abortion decision to the "medical judgment of the pregnant woman's attending physician" in the first trimester, allowing abortion to be restricted in the second trimester only in order to protect the health of the mother (i.e. by requiring that a second trimester abortion be performed in a hospital). In the third trimester, the viability of the fetus means that, unless the woman's life or health is at risk, a state can restrict abortion any way it chooses.

Although the *Roe v. Wade* decision appears to leave the abortion choice in the hands of the medical profession, the dominant legal interpretation of the decision has been that, in the first trimester, the abortion choice is essentially the woman's. This interpretation seems to be born out of the fact that while the court does require the woman's doctor to "sign off" on each abortion as proof that she had exercised her gate-keeping role, it has also defined abortion as a woman's right. It would be hard to argue that women have a right to do something if the ultimate decision about whether or not they will exercise that right rests with someone else. The interpretation of *Roe v. Wade* as granting women a right to choose was validated by another 1973 Supreme Court decision. In *Doe v. Bolton*, the Court struck down restrictive abortion laws that included requiring women to obtain permission from two doctors or a hospital committee, as a violation of both women's and doctors' rights.

Unlike the United States, the British legal system does not grant women the right to an abortion, but allows doctors to perform legal abortions in cases where an abortion is seen to be necessary. The basis of British abortion law is the Bourne decision. In 1938, Dr. Bourne performed an abortion on a fourteen-year-old girl who was pregnant as the result of a gang rape by officers of the Royal Horse Guards. One doctor had already refused to do the abortion on the grounds that the girl could be carrying the future prime minister of England. Bourne decided to operate only after he had satisfied himself that the girl was suffering such extreme nervous symptoms as a result of the rape that she was at risk of mental collapse. The jury acquitted Bourne. According to British journalist and feminist Janet Hadley, the judge on the case "compared Bourne's decision [to perform an abortion] to that of a surgeon who believes it necessary to save a patient's life by removing the appendix. If it is found that the appendix is normal—the surgeon should not be blamed, because the decision was taken 'in good faith' for the patient's welfare."[6]

This line of argument—known as the necessity defense—makes abortion legal only in circumstances where the doctor believes an abortion is necessary for the welfare of the patient. In 1967, the necessity defense was enshrined in the 1967 Abortion Act, which governs Britain, Wales, and Scotland, The Act specifies that, given the approval of two doctors, a woman may legally procure an abortion if continuing the pregnancy would threaten her life, her physical or mental health, or the physical or mental health of her existing children. Abortion is also legal if there is a "substantial risk" that the child will have serious mental or physical handicaps. According to David Nolan, the woman's environment may also be considered: "Her housing conditions, income and the support available in caring for the child, at present and in the reasonably foreseeable future."[7]

British abortion law essentially makes it the doctor's duty to ensure that women do not get abortions "on demand." The law requires doctors to act as gatekeepers, applying their own interpretation of the law and their own moral values in deciding whether or not to grant a woman's request for an abortion. Should the doctor get hauled into court for performing an abortion, a successful defense will depend on her proving that she *sincerely believed* the abortion was necessary for the welfare of her patient.

Australian abortion law also privileges the judgments of doctors over those of women. In Australia, abortion law is part of the criminal law and, as a consequence, differs from state to state. In some states, abortion is allowed because of court cases that have established "common law" precedents (Victoria, New South Wales, and Queensland). Other states have legislation that allows for abortion in specific circumstances (the Northern Territory, the Australian Capital Territory, Western Australia, and South Australia). In Tasmania, the legal status of abortion remains uncertain because there has never been a judicial test case.

Although Australia developed its own legal system decades ago, the decisions of British courts have persuasive influence. As a result, the necessity defense is the basis of both legislative and common law justifications of abortion. A recent report by the Australian National Health Medical Research Council makes it clear why the law has chosen to focus on necessity rather than women's rights: "The legal status of abortion places an obligation on doctors (and others) to play a gate-keeping role. The intention of the legislators and judge who established this role was precisely to ensure that the decision rested finally in the hands of the medical practitioner, rather than the woman."[8]

In the two most populous Australian states, Victoria and New South Wales, women must convince their practitioners that their cases fall within the guidelines developed in two legal judgments to obtain a legal abortion: the Menhennitt judgment in Victoria and the Levine ruling in New South Wales. In both cases, the judges ruled abortion could be lawful if the doctor believed on reasonable grounds that the operation was necessary to protect the woman from "a serious danger to her life or health" that the continuation of the pregnancy would entail. By danger, the judges specified that they did not mean only the physiological dangers of pregnancy and childbirth, but other physical and mental factors that might put the woman's health at risk. The judgments also specified that economic factors threatening a woman's mental or physical health could be considered as well. The Levine decision was further widened by a NSW Supreme court ruling by now High Court justice Michael Kirby in 1995. Kirby found that the woman's mental and physical health, as well as her economic situation, could be considered by the doctor, not just as they were at the time of her abortion request, but as they were likely to be after the child was born. He argued that such considerations were already a part of standard medical practice in Australia.

Despite the fact that British and Australian women's access to abortion is based on necessity, not a legal right to choose, feminist abortion activists in both countries often argue their case in terms of women's rights. A newspaper advertisement placed by the Queensland pro-choice group Children by Choice, for example, argues that abortion should be decriminalized on the grounds that "ethically and morally, it's a woman's basic right to make decisions about her own life."[9] A recent Australian study of women's experiences of abortion recommended that legal and medical practices be altered to ensure "the decision about abortion rests with women as an individual right of self determination."[10] British activist Eileen Fairweather similarly puts her pro-choice case in terms of women's rights to choose.[11] Yet despite the popularity of rights with some feminist abortion activists, other feminists believe that rights in general—and abortion rights in particular—have failed to deliver on much of their promise.

## Rights without Wrongs

The Western obsession with rights has made it difficult to see their limitations. Westerners speak of them as though they are the only moral values with meaning, and use them against each other like truncheons. When each side of the abortion debate asserts that their rights are absolute—"trumping" those claimed by their opponents—it becomes impossible to talk about ethics. As Larry Churchill and Jose Jorge Siman, teachers in the Department of Social and Administrative Medicine at the University of North Carolina, put it: "When absolute rights clash absolutely, ethics is dead in the water."[12]

One problem with the myopic obsession with rights is that we fail to recognize other important moral values, the most important of which are our responsibilities (or duties) to others. In fact, responsibilities are the counterparts to rights—you can't have one without the other. So, for example, if a fetus actually does have a right to life, in order for it to realize this right, the person *against whom* it has that right (her mother to be) must accept the responsibilities of pregnancy, birth, and parenthood. In the same way, if a woman has a right to choose an abortion, someone (in this case the wider community) is responsible for making this right a reality by, say, ensuring there are clinics that provide safe and affordable services.

Somewhere along the way, however, the responsibility side of rights got lost. Instead, rights are now seen as the absolute and private possessions of individuals, who may wield them at whim, not at the discretion of the larger community. And because the rights of one person may clash with those of another (one person's right to free speech may conflict with another's right to privacy, for example) and because no one actually gets her rights until another person accepts the responsibility for delivering them, thinking about rights individualistically ultimately leads to deadlock—with each side asserting that their rights "trump" those held by others.[13] In the abortion debate, this basically comes down to the following rather undignified argument:

ANTI-CHOICER: The fetus's right to life overrides a woman's right to control her body!

PRO-CHOICER: The woman's right to control her body trumps the fetus's right to life!

ANTI-CHOICER: Does not!

PRO-CHOICER: Does too!

ANTI-CHOICER: Does not!

PRO-CHOICER: Does too . . .

Each side wants it all, and neither wants to give anything; and so the argument goes around and around with the rules of the game effectively ruling out compromise.

The individualistic way we think about rights has also led many feminists to adopt a give-me-my-rights-and-then-butt-out attitude in the abortion debate. Say Churchill and Siman:

Both sides of the abortion debate have succumbed to an individualistic rights rhetoric . . . feminists have neglected their social roots, and do not see themselves as belonging in any fundamental way to the community. Hence they treat their bodies and their reproductive capacities as private property and regard any suggestion of obligation as an infringement. Right-to-life advocates generally do not think they belong in any real sense to a community either. Their advocacy for the fetus is grounded in a self-serving and fragmented notion of life. Fetal life is valued and protected, but the obligation to support the newborn, adolescent, or adult life is absent.[14]

Janet Hadley has worried that feminist enthusiasm for this individualistic notion of rights has given the public the false impression that aborting women are irresponsible:

"It's my right" is an individualist stance, relying on autonomy, privacy and bodily integrity to defy any outside scrutiny or comment. So when defenders of abortion wear badges declaring "Get your laws off our bodies," they may inadvertently bolster the pernicious portrayal of women who have abortions as doing so for no more reasons than their own feckless whim and shallow "convenience."[15]

A final problem with rights, says British legal academic Carol Smart, is that while they are formulated to protect the weak from the powerful, they often end up being used by the powerful at the expense of the weak. For instance, while sex discrimination legislation was intended as a tool for women to remedy historical inequities in areas like employment, housing, and medical care, men have begun using such laws to argue that gender-specific initiatives—like women's health programs—discriminate against *them*. In her maiden speech to the Australian parliament in 1996, independent MP Pauline Hanson invoked the Racial Discrimination Act to argue that assistance programs for Aboriginal people discriminate against her because she is white: "Today . . . I talk about . . . the privileges Aboriginals enjoy over other Australians. I have done research on benefits only available to Aboriginals and challenge anyone to tell me how Aboriginals are disadvantaged when they can obtain 3 and 5 percent housing loans denied to non-Aboriginals.

(While the facts were clearly irrelevant to the put-upon Ms. Hanson, it is worth pointing out that while disadvantaged Aboriginal people are able to get loans fixed at 2 to 5 percent for the first year and capped at 8 percent thereafter, this scheme is similar to those run in a number of states for low-income earners, and to schemes for defense force personnel.)

## The Value of Rights and the Specter of Maternal Duty

Despite their problems, many feminists have strenuously objected to a withdrawal from the rights position staked out by the pro-choice movement. They argue that because rights are our culture's primary moral currency, making a claim in the language of rights gives the claim legitimacy. It also, according to Carol Smart, makes the claim comprehensible and accessible to everyone: "To pose an issue in terms of rights [means] it enters into a linguistic currency to which everyone has access. Moreover, whilst the extension of rights is associated with the foundations of democracy and freedom, the claim to rights is always already loaded. It is almost as hard to be against rights as it is to be against virtue."[16]

In addition, while many feminists know that rights are not perfect, they are at a loss to come up with an alternative that isn't even *more* oppressive to women. Smart, for example, rules out returning to the days when women seeking abortion were "unfortunates" in need of "rescue":

With . . . abortion rights, the women's movement . . . transform[ed] the politics of abortion from a benevolent response to the "plight" of unfortunate women, to a question of legitimate rights that should apply to all women. Although the "plight" imagery has not faded completely, it has been a measure of political success that matters which were once the focus of charitable works are now questions of adequate provision to meet legitimate demand. The problem with abandoning the rights discourse is that the image of the desperate woman returns . . . The fear is that women may have to sacrifice their dignity in the area of abortion if we abandon rights.[17]

Even as brilliant a feminist thinker as Rosalind Petchesky has trouble envisioning a non–rights-based approach to reproductive choice that remains true to feminist values:

We should pursue the discourse now begun towards developing a feminist ethic of reproductive freedom that complements feminist politics. What ought we to choose if we became genuinely free to choose? Are some choices unacceptable on moral grounds, and does this mean under any circumstances, or only under some? Can feminism reconstruct a joyful sense of childbearing and maternity without capitulating to ideologies that reduce women to a maternal essence? Can we talk about morality in reproductive decision-making without invoking the spectre of maternal duty?[18]

Because the idea of maternal responsibility is such a minefield for feminists, Janet Hadley has gone so far as to conclude that the current political climate around abortion precludes the feminist movement articulating a feminist abortion morality that argues for anything other than a woman's right to choose:

> Questioning the morality of the reasons women have abortions is a minefield for feminism. When for the forseeable future childrearing is going to remain the province of mothers, it seems impossible to challenge a woman's decision to have an abortion without invoking something smacking of "maternal duty." That is why almost all feminist advocacy of women's rights to abortion in an unjust world centers on her right to decide, that is, the politics, and not the reasons for her decision.[19]

So what is "maternal duty," and why are feminists so scared of it? Maternal duty is really shorthand for the ideology around motherhood that asserts that a "good" mother is a natural with children, puts her children's needs before her own and makes motherhood her main occupation (at least when her children are small). I'll talk more about the ideology of "good motherhood" in chapter 5 and for the moment restrict myself to explaining why feminists get so itchy when motherhood and responsibility are mentioned in the same sentence. In my view, it is because feminists have worked so hard to convince society, and women themselves, that the capacity for self-sacrifice is not an essential—nor even a desirable—attribute of a "good" mother or a "good" woman. It was the feminist movement that sought to "raise" women's consciousness about their own needs as people and to encourage them to seek ways to meet those needs. While for some women this meant balancing their childcare responsibilities with work, for others it meant demanding that their partners share in the housework and childcare. Essentially, it allowed women to focus not only on their responsibilities to others but on their own rights to happiness and fulfillment.

Yet, while feminists rightly fear a return to the days when mothering was all about responsibility and self-sacrifice and being a woman was all about mothering, many also seem convinced that an ideal feminist abortion morality should emphasize both women's rights and their responsibilities. British feminists Lynda Birke, Susan Himmelweit, and Gail Vines, for instance, allude to the importance of responsibility when they reject an approach to women's reproductive freedom that is solely focused on rights:

We do not feel that a "reproductive rights" approach . . . is adequate. In particular, we feel that it tends to make it impossible to discuss the reasons why women make particular reproductive decisions. Having said that it is a woman's right to choose seems to leave little room for any further discussion. But, in practice, it is still possible to say that, from a feminist point of view, some reasons for aborting a fetus are good ones, for example, if a woman does not feel ready to be a mother, while others, for example, that she wants only to give her husband a son, are bad ones.[20]

Regis Dunne, a member of the Australian National Bioethics Consultative Committee, believes that a true moral perspective involves asking and answering more questions than "Do I have a right to do this?": "The argument that the persons involved are acting freely and exercising their liberty does not take into account whether in the overall public good they are entitled to do this, as the consequences will not be contained with them, nor does it address the moral question of whether they ought to do this."[21]

## Feminists and Morality

While they have been enthusiastic about rights, most feminists have sought to separate pro-choice arguments from questions of morality. Their major concern has been—and continues to be—that making abortion a moral issue opens women up for inappropriate judgment by others. What if allowing women to be judged *morally* wanting in regard to abortion leads to their being *legally* denied a termination? In the United Kingdom and Australia, where abortion is still technically illegal, this worry has particular potency.

Part of the strategy feminists have used to drive a wedge between morality and the abortion issue is to question anti choice assertions that they hold the moral high ground—or any moral ground at all—in the debate. Feminists have pointed out, for example, the fact that anti-choicers push to re-criminalize abortion despite the fact that the disastrous consequences for women in making abortion illegal are well known. One study of New York women who'd had a safe and legal abortion found that 45 percent would have tried to get an abortion even if it was illegal. Globally, an estimated 13 percent of pregnancy-related deaths—or one in eight—are the result of unsafe abortion. While 700,000 women die each year from unsafe abortions, much larger numbers experience a range of complications, which include sepsis, hemorrhage, uterine perforation, kidney failure, and even coma. A South African study of 647 women hospitalized after unsafe abortions found that 35 had to have a hysterectomy. Eighteen of those losing their uterus had never had children, and eight were under the age of twenty. How moral is it, feminists have rightly asked, to make abortion illegal when it has been shown, time and time again, that it leads to the involvement of organized crime in abortions, and heaps of women dying or becoming infertile from backyard abortions?

Feminists have also asked how moral it is to support recriminalization when this results in the birth of more unwanted—and so at-risk—children. Eight out of ten babies murdered by their mothers, for example, are from unwanted pregnancies. In addition, studies have found that unwanted children have more insecure childhoods, receive more psychiatric care, and are at greater risk of delinquency.[22] One woman tells her story of being unwanted this way:

I often ask myself if the people demonstrating [against abortion] know what it means to be an unwanted child. My mother committed suicide when I was three and my father rejected me because I wasn't born a boy. I was a desperately lonely and unloved child. When my father remarried several years later I clung to little bits of affection occasionally tossed my way by my stepmother. Most of the time, she rejected me too. There is no doubt in my mind that it would have been better for me not to have been born. My mother should have aborted me.[23]

In the United States, the feminist rejection of the moral had a strong connection to the anti-choice religious right's promotion of itself as the "moral" voice of the Republican movement. The agenda of the Christian right is, to put it rather baldly, to make the Bible (rather than the secular U.S. Constitution) the supreme law of the land. The United States religious right, like most religious extremists, believe that their political views are actually God's will. This means that those opposing them are simply seen as wrong, godless, and immoral. Rather than question the religious right's assertions that support for budget cuts to the poor, elderly, and disabled is moral, feminists joined with other groups (like the American Civil Liberties Union) in protesting the Republican party's complete disregard of the separation between church and state. One of the unfortunate side effects of this strategy was the perception that feminism was opposed to morality itself, rather than to one religious group's imposition of its rather narrow version of morality on a pluralistic society. Unfortunately, the arrogant belief of anti-choice supporters that they have exclusive knowledge of the moral is not confined to the United States. In response to an article I wrote in Melbourne's *Age* newspaper on pro-choice abortion ethics, one anti-choicer had this to say: "Get real! How can adoption be a more painful experience than abortion? It is the termination of a potent living future. The universal psyche already carries enough grief and sadness without these pro-choicers thinking they can honourably add to it."[24] Finally, many feminists have been wary of bringing ethics into the abortion debate because they know it means taking a long, hard look at their relationship with the fetus.

## The Fetus

In the early days of the abortion struggle, feminist arguments about abortion didn't so much put women at their center as put women in *by themselves*. Feminists would contend that getting an abortion was no different from getting a haircut or a tonsillectomy, that the fetus was just a "clump of cells" or the equivalent of a fish. In the United States, abortion was asserted to be a "health issue, not a moral issue," while rallying U.K. feminists chanted: "An egg is not a chicken, an acorn is not a tree, a fetus is not a baby, so don't lay that on me." While feminists had wisely realized that it was impossible for two sets of rights—the fetus's and the woman's—to be contained in one set of skin, they had not only rejected fetal rights, but the fetus itself (a case of throwing the baby out with the bath water, so to speak). In addition, the inexperience of the women's movement led to early feminist abortion politics being mostly reactive.

British feminist Eileen Fairweather, writing in the radical feminist rag *Spare Rib*, tells how this caused both the reality of the fetus and women's experience of abortion to drop out of feminist abortion politics:

> The women's movement was still very young when abortion first became a political football. We duly kicked back and, faced with the opposition's set of slogans, defensively came up with our own. In our rush to do that, the complexity of abortion and its emotional significance for women somehow got lost . . . Our opponents prey upon the emotional effects of abortion, so we play them down . . . they talk of killing life, and speak of every foetus as a baby. In response . . . [we] say "the foetus is a potential human life, incapable of independent existence . . ."[25]

Pro-choice wariness of the fetus also has its roots in the anti-choice movement's misuse of fetal bodies and parts to score cheap political points. Fetal-flashing—displaying or shoving a fetus into well-known pro-choicers' hands—has long been a staple publicity-generator for those on the fringe of the anti-choice movement. But with the disintegration of the coalition of conservative interests that led to Bill Clinton's defeat of George Bush in the 1992 U.S. presidential election, a desperate and increasingly marginalized anti-choice movement has increased its use of such tactics. When Clinton was stumping in New York during the 1992 election campaign, he was stalked by an anti-choice woman and her boyfriend, who waited in the crowds with a fetus in a plastic bag. When the woman waited so long that she missed the "right moment" to spring the fetus on the candidate, she didn't give up. Instead, she threw the fetus at him. Joe Scheidler, founder of the Pro-Life Action League, averred that the installation of a pro-choice president in the White House did not spell the end of "fetal flashing": "When Clinton got elected, we didn't close shop. [He] will have to view dead babies for his four years, or eight, or whatever. We're going to make sure of that."[26]

The pro-choice movement has been quick to condemn fetal-flashing as "extreme" and "ghoulish," pointing out that, despite anti-choice claims to the contrary, the vast majority of fetuses being flashed are closer to twenty-two weeks than twelve. This approach, however, does little to dispel the suspicion of those who watch such antics, and the leader of anti-choice Operation Rescue, Keith Tucci, may have a point when he says that "showing a dead fetus is not gory, making dead fetuses is gory."[27]

The real problem with fetal-flashing is not its "ghastliness" but its complete unhinging of the contextual moorings that make most women's abortions both comprehensible and justifiable. It is because the context is missing that the anti-choice movement gets away with flashing fetuses that in most cases are still-born, not aborted, and most likely have parents who would be both injured and outraged if they knew how their dead fetuses were being used. If the attitudes of the women I interviewed are a trustworthy guide, the women whose aborted fetuses were being misused in this way would be similarly outraged. The following conversation, between myself, Lisa, Carey, and Lucy, began after I raised the question of medical science's use of fetal tissue to treat those suffering from Parkinson's disease:

CAREY: Are they telling the people who have abortions?

LC: I don't know. They might be, I'm not sure.

LUCY: If you had actually had an abortion, would you actually say no? There was this woman, she was totally incapacitated with Parkinson's and she got 80 percent of all her functions back . . .

CAREY: I'm not saying I'd say no, I'm just saying that you have to ask the woman if it's OK to use the aborted tissue!

LUCY: But if it's in the rubbish bin, if she's just thinking it's going in the bin . . .

LISA: But you can't take it home, can you?

LUCY: You can't take it home, and they can use it . . . It has been created especially for science to use.

CAREY: I think that is outrageous, absolutely outrageous . . . Not even asking permission.

LUCY: But still, it's like they're taking out your appendix and throwing it in the rubbish. You're throwing it in the rubbish, you haven't said you want it all prettied up and put in a nice grave and buried.

LISA: No way, they can't just take it.

LUCY: OK, but your actual appendix is diced out, and the fetus is diced out. It's out of you, it's not part of you. I mean it's gone, you've chosen to murder. You've killed that child, it's gone.

LISA: If they're doing stuff like that, I'm going to start taking my tupperware container with me.

CAREY: Oh, absolutely.

LC: So you think you have a right to the fetus, even if you've just "tossed it in the bin"?

CAREY: The whole handling of the abortion issue is wrong. You don't toss it in the garbage. I mean, I've had an abortion, it was an incredibly painful experience. I didn't toss it in the garbage. And I find it really distressing to hear it referred to in that way. And that others think they have a right to use my fetus. You're saying toss it in the garbage. I didn't toss it in the garbage.

LC: OK, what did you do?

CAREY: It sounds very callous and my decision was not a callous one. It was not unthought about, it was not clear, and it certainly wasn't indifferent. Part of your abortion decision is that it's not going to be used as fetal tissue [to treat disease] or anything else. The thing is that if somebody asked me could it be used as fetal tissue, I'd probably say yes. But not to ask . . .

The story and reasons of the aborting woman unknown, the fetus found in a plastic bag in a dumpster is seen to be as alone and abandoned as a half-grown Christmas puppy. The supposed indifference of the fetus's mother is then handily contrasted with the intense concern of those in the anti-choice movement. "We Care" asserts many a banner in anti-choice protest marches. Janet Hadley has noted that the most successful strategy has been the presentation of the anti-choice movement as representing the "only people with any sense of concern about the fetus."[28]

The anti-choice movement doesn't only misuse fetal bodies, it manipulates and misuses fetal images. The Western tradition privileges what we see with our eyes. Seeing, in other words, is believing, as an anti-choice bumper sticker that exhorts us to "Visualize the Fetus!" demonstrates. Accordingly, the anti-choice movement has worked hard to make the fetus a visible public presence by "littering the background of any abortion talk" with

chaste silhouettes of the fetal form, or voyeuristic-necrophilist photographs of its remains. These still images float like spirits through the courtrooms, where lawyers argue that foetuses can claim tort liability, through the hospital and clinics, where physicians welcome them as "patients," and in front of all the abortion centers, legislative committees, bus terminals and other places "right-to-lifers" haunt.[29]

The fantastic images of fetuses in utero obtainable with high-tech photographic equipment, ultrasounds, and magnetic resonance imaging give the deceptive impression of the fetus as a cosmonaut, an independent and self-contained unit floating around in "space." These technologies build an image of the fetus—one in defiance of the facts—as a miniature person *who just happens* to reside inside a woman's body. Barbara Rothman, an American bioethicist who has extensively researched women's experience of pre-natal testing procedures like amniocentesis, observes:

These new images of the fetus and even the embryo are making us aware of the "unborn" . . . but they do so at the cost of making the mother transparent. Picture to yourself the photos you have seen of fetuses in utero, wriggling, sucking their tiny fingers. Where did they lie in their mothers? Where was that fetus in relation to her body, to her navel, her heart, her pelvis? It existed as if in space. Indeed, the fetus in utero has become a metaphor for "man" in space, floating free, attached only by the umbilical cord of the spaceship. But where is the mother in that metaphor? She has become empty space.[30]

Rosalind Petchesky takes this idea one step further:

The [image of] the autonomous, free-floating foetus merely extends to gestation the Hobbesian view of born human beings as disconnected, solitary individuals . . . this abstract individualism, effacing the pregnant woman and the fetus' dependence on her, [lets us] read in it ourselves, our lost babies, our mythic secure past.[31]

Of course, seeing is not the only way of knowing about a pregnancy if you happen to be the woman who is pregnant. As British sociologist Anne Oakley has pointed out: "Women cannot see into their own wombs, but . . . generally have some idea what is going on in them."[32] Nonetheless, the centerpiece of anti-choice propaganda, the equation of the fetus with the baby, depends on our culture's faith in the "truth" of what is seen. The anti-choice argument is mostly made up of photographs that attempt to reduce the development process of a human being to a single image that the public will respond to like it was a newborn baby. The equation of a four-celled embryo or a deaf, blind, translucent and microscopic fetus with a newborn baby, however, is not easy. Celeste Condit, a feminist and a specialist in the creation of political rhetoric, explains how the anti-choice movement has successfully doctored and mislabelled images of the fetus to make powerful arguments for their cause:

> The process is necessarily one of reduction—the creation of a simple label or name for a whole entity from *visible* attributes or associations. In the abortion case the wide variety of beings that constitute developing unborn human life-forms—the blastocyst, embryo, fetus, viable baby—were reduced to a single entity through the creation of a single vision of the "unborn baby."[33]

In order for the anti-choice movement to persuade the public to see images of even extremely young fetuses as no different from those of the newborn baby, it needed to widely disseminate

> pictures of a fetus in the third or late-second trimester. In the pictures, the fetus was largely independent of its placenta and umbilical cord. The photographs featured no blood or placental tissue to turn stomachs queasy, they focus on head and feet . . . When pictures of younger fetuses appeared, they were either prominently labeled "baby, surrounded by older fetuses and by babies, or accompanied by text that attributed baby-like features to them (e.g. thumb-sucking, heartbeat, brain activity).[34]

Condit tells how anti-choice activists are specifically instructed to "begin their slide shows with a picture of a baby and work backward in development to establish the continuity of life forms."[35] Only in this way could the indistinguishable embryo be "seen" as a baby. The pro-choice movement has decided not to specifically counter such anti-choice visuals with ones of their own (one feminist has suggested placards with pictures of "bloody, lumpy early-term abortions or unenhanced early-term sonograms").[36] Consequently, the fetus = baby equation continues to gain ground.

Yet the denial of the reality and importance of the fetus—a denial that runs counter to the experience of many women—has wound up backfiring on the pro-choice movement. Not only have pro-choice women been "denied access" to the fetus because of the implicit understanding that it was the property of the other side, the pro-choice movement's reluctance to engage with the fetus has been used as evidence of feminist heartlessness.

## Feminists of a Different Stripe

Over the years, there have been a few feminists who noticed—and even complained—about the absence of the fetus in the pro-choice side of the abortion debate. Although I didn't find her on the NOW bookshelves, Linda Bird Francke began raising ethical concerns about the feminist approach to abortion back in 1978. Kathleen McDonnell's book *Not an Easy Choice: A Feminist Re-examines Abortion* appeared in 1984. Both women made a plea for allowing the fetus, and morality, into the feminist position on abortion.

Francke's first contact with what she called the "ambivalence" of abortion began in 1976 (three years after abortion was made legal in America), when she wrote in the *New York Times* about her own abortion. Thirty-eight years old, the last of her three children just starting school, Francke was looking forward to returning to the workforce she had all but abandoned to raise her children. Her husband was also hoping to change to a more interesting, but less secure, job. Then she became pregnant. Were these good enough reasons to have an abortion? Francke wasn't sure. Despite her ambivalence, she went ahead with the abortion, and she and her husband returned to their lives. At the end of the piece, Francke affirms her abortion choice, yet reflects on the guilt she continues to feel for not choosing to "make room" in her life for another child. Francke's story struck a cord among the readers of the *New York Times*. Letters from pro's, anti's and those in between came pouring in. The nascent anti-choice movement—after removing a few sentences that didn't suit—sent Francke's article to everyone on their mailing list.

Perhaps it was Francke's experience of being so rudely appropriated by the other side that led Kathleen McDonnell to take such a tentative tone in *Not an Easy Choice*. Certainly McDonnell worried in the chapter entitled "Morality and Abortion" that even recognizing the moral dimensions of the abortion issue could give "ammunition" to abortion opponents. She claimed, however, that because most people have a "gut feeling that abortion *is* a moral issue," the willingness of the anti-choice movement to address the

moral dimensions of abortion, however simplistically, was attracting even those who found their views too extreme.

Despite their efforts, neither Francke's nor McDonnell's books
had much impact on the way the pro-choice case was argued by the
feminist movement, most likely because neither was able to propose
a coherent alternative to the rights-based approach that didn't risk
compromising women's integrity or freedom. So, a little over ten
years after *Not an Easy Choice* was published, another feminist
tried to wake the movement to the moral dimensions of the abortion issue. Her name was Naomi Wolf, and her stature unfortunately guaranteed that her somewhat incoherent views on the subject would garner a great deal of attention.

Wolf became the youthful darling of the American feminist
scene after the publication of her book, *The Beauty Myth*. She
dropped out of public view to have her first child about the time
her second book, *Fire with Fire*, was failing to ignite the same sort
of media attention—or sales—*The Beauty Myth* had enjoyed. At
the end of 1995 she put her hat into the abortion ring with a piece
in the *New Republic*. Wolf's opinion was that feminism had failed
to listen to women and had lost "mainstream" American voter support by refusing to recognize abortion as a moral issue in which the
fetus is an important player. So far so good. Wolf then argued that
the only way for the pro-choice movement to regain this support
was to adopt her "paradigm of sin and redemption." What this
paradigm boils down to is three simple—if not simplistic—propositions. They are:

- All abortions are wrong.
- Women have a right to choose abortion.
- Women are sinners when they have an abortion.

According to Wolf, a woman "redeems" her abortion "sin" when
she "face[s] the realization that she has fallen short of who she
should be, and . . . ask[s] forgiveness for that, and atone[s] for it."[37]

Leaving aside Wolf's curious decision to resuscitate such medie-
val notions as sin and redemption, a bigger problem for Wolf's theory is the contention that, because many women feel badly about

abortion, abortion is morally wrong. Certainly it is true that some women do feel badly about having an abortion, but so too do they feel badly about having a child they are unable to support, or a child they must put up for adoption. Does that mean these choices are also "sins"? According to the National Academy of Sciences in Washington, D.C., there is "probably no psychologically painless way to cope with an unwanted pregnancy." Wolf is also wrong to suppose that if a woman feels badly about abortion she therefore believes she did the wrong thing. Jojo's response to her abortion on this count is typical: "I was brought up a Catholic and it's a no-no to have an abortion [but] I couldn't handle having a baby at the moment . . . I'm really glad I had the abortion."[38]

Wolf's belief that abortion is an "evil" practice may please a few hard-line Catholics but many religious groups refuse to issue such simplistic moral absolutes. Numerous religions—Quakers, some Methodist sects, Judaism, Islam—hold that not only is abortion permitted in some circumstances, it is morally required.[39] According to Janet Hadley, some Japanese Buddhists allow abortion, believing that too many children weaken the family unit and that unwanted children are a tragedy. Wolf talks endlessly about trivial, selfish women—including herself in a former life—who have trivial, selfish abortions. She quotes extensively from the story of a woman named Redman in an attempt to "demonstrate" that Redman has a callous—and typically feminist—attitude toward abortion. Wolf describes how Redman

schedules her chemical abortion. The procedure is experimental and [Redman] feels "almost heroic" thinking of how she is blazing a trail for other women . . . Redman is on a *Woman's Day* march when the blood from the abortion first appears. She exults at this: "Our bodies, our lives, our right to decide . . . my life feels luxuriant with possibility. For one precious moment, I believe that we have the power to dismantle this system. I finish the march, borne along by the women.[40]

In addition to supporting the bid (already quite successful, thank you very much) of the anti-choice movement to depict feminists as cold, self-centered baby-and-mother haters, academic Rebecca Albury believes that the Redman story provides essential support for Wolf's underlying argument: that what a "silly and flighty" woman needs is "a lesson that 24 hour responsibility for a child would provide."[41]

Albury believes that the problem with the "my body, my choice" approach is a mismatch between feminist rhetoric and women's experiences: "A foetus is not carried around as if hidden in the boot of a car for nine months; a woman is pregnant. She feels the growing foetus and conducts her life among people who expect pregnant women to become mothers."[42]

The point is that women don't *own* their bodies (as they own the boot of their car), they *are* their bodies. Pregnant women aren't the same people with a few extra kilos strapped to their middles; they are becoming—to themselves and for others—different people. Not only does the rhetoric of body ownership ignore women's experiences of pregnancy, it makes it difficult for feminists to explain why some of the things women do with their bodies feel so wrong. After all, if it is "hers," why can't she do with it what she likes?

This conundrum stymies feminist attempts to talk about morality when it comes to abortion. In the middle of 1996, there was a furor in Britain after a young single mother, pregnant again with twins, decided to abort one fetus because she "was too poor" to raise both. The pro-choice response to this case—supporters insisted it was no different from any other abortion—was unsatisfyingly terse and decidedly unpersuasive. In the same way, feminists have been left without the language or the concepts to question the trend that encourages women to abort fetuses that are—or may be—damaged. Many disabled people worry that such abortions (always supported and in some instances promoted by the medical profession) further devalue the disabled in society and may lead ultimately to the refusal of governments to support families who "choose" to have a disabled baby. The "right to choose" concept is also of little help when it comes to explaining why the practice of female infanticide, practiced across much of Asia, is so morally repugnant. Feminists Lynda Birke, Susan Himmelweit, and Gail Vines sum up the problem: "A problem with the 'right to choose' is that the choices made by individuals may have social effects that are undesirable. Not only are individuals' choices always made within an economic, cultural and political context, but that context is itself affected by the decisions of individuals."[43]

## Mainstreaming versus Morality

The bottom line for all feminists is the same—to ensure that all women (regardless of where they live and how much money they have) have access to safe and legal abortions. North American abortion clinic violence has left North American feminists in search of effective strategies—both theoretical and practical—to keep adequate numbers of abortion clinics open for business. The strategy most of them have chosen is the mainstreaming of abortion provision into other health services for women. Burying women's abortion services in mainstream medical clinics goes hand in hand with redefining abortion from being an ethical issue to a health issue. This is explained by Rick Hudson:

> I feel very strongly that abortion services must be mainstreamed as part of a policy package of dealing with unintended pregnancy . . . I was disappointed . . . that [the Australian National Health and Medical Research Council's report on abortion] didn't take a clear stand that abortion is a routine health service . . . In British Columbia we have . . . a women's health center that do[es] terminations within a large hospital campus. [It] has never been subject to harassment, yet the two free-standing clinics have been constantly harassed. Though free-standing abortion clinics represent a commitment to women's health, when you mainstream abortion as part of a general women's health [service] you get a principle of diffusion. If you diffuse something it can't be a target.[44]

Although Hudson doesn't mention it, part of the "diffusion" approach involves supporting the development of "abortion pills" like RU 486. The hope is that women may one day be prescribed abortions the same way they are currently prescribed penicillin—by prescription from their general practitioner.[45]

The main problem with the abortion-as-just-another-women's-health-need approach is more principled than practical. The reality is that women are facing real danger in procuring abortions in North America, and doctors face real physical danger in providing them. If tucking clinics away in other facilities and promoting drugs like RU 486 is necessary to protect physical health and safety, then so be it (with the caveat that all abortion drugs need to be tested before they are freely dispensed to women).[46] The problem is that

moving abortion services to mainstream medical facilities supports
the definition of abortion as a routine health requirement, rather
than a woman's issue with complex ethical, medical, and social implications. Once women have abortions for health reasons, all those
performed for non-therapeutic purposes are seen as "discretionary"
and therefore "frivolous." Even if the grounds for a "medical"
abortion are construed broadly enough to take in a woman's mental, emotional, and physical health, defining abortion as a medical
issue denies and disguises the complexity of women's reproductive
choices. Such complexity must be acknowledged if a case for the
moral nature of most women's abortion choices is to be made.

Once abortions are classified as either "justified" or "unjus-
tified" (and women as either "deserving" or "undeserving"), abortion reverts to being a secret and shameful event for women. In addition, medical abortions deny women's moral agency and their
capacity to make their own choices, based on their own values.
Says Rosalind Petchesky: "Medical . . . models of abortion . . .
focus . . . on 'hardship' situations—rubella, rape, mental illness—
and thus 'always picture . . . women as victims . . . never as possible
shapers of their own destinies' . . . These models implicitly suggest
. . . that women [are] incompetent to act as moral agents on their
own behalf . . ."[47]

My point is that while there are clearly practical and tactical ad-
vantages in de-emphasizing the moral content, and thus the "special" and often medical nature of the abortion decision, it is possible that what women gain in their capacity to more readily access
safe and legal abortions, they may lose in their ability to see themselves, and be seen by others, as the final source of moral decision-
making about abortion. Ultimately, insisting upon women's moral
agency in abortion may be just as critical to securing women's abortion freedoms as is reducing their physical vulnerability at abortion
clinics.

•  •  •

While there are clearly some abortions that make feminists distinctly uncomfortable, the language of rights, and the belief that the
only wrong in abortion lies in denying a woman the freedom to

have one, makes it difficult for them to say why. The moral vacuum left by the pro-choice movement has not only been filled by the distorted images of fetuses promulgated by the anti-choice movement, and by the technological "solutions" to the abortion problem proposed by ethicists like Singer and Wells, but by the inflexible moral language of absolute rights. While it is clear that reclaiming the moral ground in the debate will require making space for the fetus, the next chapter vividly demonstrates how important it is to remember that, first and foremost, that space is always inside a woman.

# · 3 ·

# The Downward Spiral of Viability and the Urgent Need for Change

I'm like a lot of people. I'm in the mushy middle.
—NORMA McCORVEY

In 1969, a twenty-one-year-old Texas single mother of two named Norma McCorvey discovered she was pregnant. Abortion was illegal in Texas and McCorvey didn't have the money to travel to a state where it was legal. In the end, she had the baby and gave it up for adoption. McCorvey's case—which challenged the constitutionality of laws prohibiting abortion—eventually wound up in the Supreme Court. The *Roe v. Wade* decision that was handed down in 1973 granted American women the right to choose abortion and made McCorvey (a.k.a. Jane Roe) a potent symbol of the pro-choice movement. In 1995, when McCorvey—now a born-again Christian—announced she was no longer sure where she stood on the abortion issue, the pro-choice movement went into a tailspin.

The problem was that McCorvey's move was a visible symbol of the slide of Americans away from the pro-choice movement even as substantial numbers continued—in opinion polls—to express support for a woman's right to choose. Slippage in the numbers is not a phenomenon confined to the United States. While over three-quarters of Australians believe the abortion decision should be left to the individual and her doctor, support for the pro-choice position has waned since its high point in the early 1990s. In 1991, 81 percent of Australians favored freedom of choice, and this number had dropped to 77 percent by 1996. Particularly worrying is the desertion of the pro-choice movement by the young. A 1995 Morgan Gallup poll found that only 51 percent of Australians aged fourteen to twenty-four supported choice, while among those aged fifty and over, support for choice was at 56 percent.

• • •

Cornelia Whitner has been serving an eight-year sentence in a South Carolina jail for using cocaine during pregnancy. In the most recent ruling on the case, the South Caroline Supreme Court held that a viable fetus is a "person," and that even though her son was born healthy, Whitner had "endangered [his] life, health and comfort." In addition to Whitner, up to four other women are currently serving out long sentences for "fetal abuse" in South Carolina jails.[1]

The focus on individual women who "abuse" their fetuses continues to dominate the news in the United States. In the media frenzies surrounding such cases, those who try to douse the flames by placing such tragedies into context are shunned (feminists typically note the refusal of drug-and-alcohol treatment programs to accept pregnant women; the fact that almost all women arrested for fetal "crimes" are poor and non-white; and the lack of social and financial support systems available to single mothers). Successful prosecution of Whitner's case, and others like it, relies on the medical "fact" of viability. Prosecutors either assume or seek to prove that there is no difference between a viable fetus and a child that has been born—a baby. Once judges, juries, and society in general accept that there are no important differences between a fetus and a baby, endowing the fetus with the same legal rights as a baby is the logical next step. From there, successful prosecution of "abusive" pregnant women is pretty much in the bag. After all, if a *child*-abusing woman deserves to be punished, why not a *fetus*-abusing one? The question, of course, is whether a fetus really is the same as a baby. Or to ask the same question differently, is the pregnant woman's relationship with her fetus exactly the same as her relationship with her child?

• • •

On March 22, [1996,] a Florida Court found that a low-income woman who shot herself in the stomach in her sixth month of pregnancy could be prosecuted for manslaughter but not third-degree murder. The woman, Kawana Ashley, was a nineteen-year-old single mother of a three-year-old who was living with her grandmother when she became pregnant. Although she knew that she could not support a second child, she was unable to obtain an abortion because the Florida Medicaid program—her sole source of health care—only covers the procedure in cases of life endangerment, rape or incest. Her fetus, which was only grazed by the bullet, died shortly after from complications of prematurity.[2]

As in the Whitner case, those prosecuting Kawana Ashley were convinced of the importance—and the factual nature—of viability and fetal personhood. But the actual point at which a fetus is viable is *not* a hard medical fact. A fetus that is viable in New York City, for instance, may not be viable in Pakistan. Why? For the simple reason that, in Pakistan, the expensive and high-tech equipment needed to preserve the fetus just isn't available.

The skill and interest of medical centers and particular medical specialists in saving extremely premature babies is also a vital factor in determining viability. There are whispers, for instance, that while the neo-natal team at Melbourne's Monash Medical Centre will pull out all the stops to save any baby born alive, the Royal Children's Hospital takes a more restrained approach. In addition, fetuses of the same gestational age have highly variable survival rates. Only one-third of fetuses born at twenty-eight weeks, for example, are developed enough to survive.

More important, whether a fetus is or is not a person is a question of *value*, not of fact. Viability, in other words, is as arbitrary a place to draw a line between fetushood and personhood as is conception—where the Pope draws it—or birth. Other dividing lines proposed have been quickening (when the woman feels the fetus move), implantation (when the fertilized embryo becomes embedded in the wall of its mother's uterus), and the time when the "primitive streak" appears in the embryo (distinguishing which cluster of cells will become the fetus and which the placenta). The point is

# SOME FACTS ABOUT FETAL VIABILITY

Currently, even fetuses in technologically advanced countries only become viable late in the second trimester, or at about the twenty-fourth week of pregnancy. So while those who express concerns about fetal viability currently have little to worry about (fewer than about 2.5 percent of all abortions take place after this time), the anti-choice movement has sought to use public disquiet with the rare second-trimester abortion, and with some second-trimester abortion techniques, to undermine support for women's access to abortions at earlier stages of pregnancy.

## The United States

Feminist joy at the respect shown to women by the United States Supreme Court in granting them the right to choose in *Roe v. Wade* has been dampened in recent times by growing feminist realization that the emphasis the decision places on fetal viability to uphold its trimester framework is a time bomb that could explode in women's faces. No less prominent a figure that Justice Sandra Day O'Connor, the first female justice to sit in the Court, has recognized this fact. In her 1983 dissent from the *Akron v. Akron Center for Reproductive Health* decision—one that largely reaffirmed a woman's right to be free from "undue burdens" from state laws when choosing abortion—O'Connor pointed out that improvements in medical science were pushing the point of viability further back, toward conception, expanding the time period in which *Roe v. Wade* allows states to regulate or prohibit abortion. The *Roe v. Wade* decision, she said, "was on a collision course with itself." In 1989, the Court upheld the right of the State of Missouri to find that "the life of each human being begins at conception" and to require any woman who appeared more than twenty-two weeks pregnant to submit to tests to determine the viability of the fetus.

The 1992 decision in *Planned Parenthood v. Casey* was at the very least a "technical victory" for pro-choice forces, retaining the essence of *Roe v. Wade* by affirming a woman's right to choose abortion before viability.[3] But the decision also offered something to anti-choice forces in its sanctioning of four of the five restrictions on women's choice described by Pennsylvania law. It also, according to Janet Hadley, implicitly sanctioned states creating "a further raft of restrictions, provided they did not impose an undue burden on a woman seeking abortion. The criteria for an undue burden appeared to be something that a well-heeled middle-class woman would not find too irksome."[4]

Concerns about viability may also affect the decision a U.S. doctor makes about the abortion procedure he uses, because the states are empowered to require a physician to use the abortion method most likely to result in fetal survival if it does not pose a significantly greater health risk to the woman. States can also require the attendance of a second physician at post-viability procedures to take control of the fetus if it is born alive.[5]

## Britain

While the 1967 British Abortion Act makes no specific reference to any upper time limits for abortions, it does refer to an earlier piece of legislation—the Infant Life (Preservation) Act of 1929—in which the destruction of a child "capable of being born alive" was prohibited. While many believed that this meant that no abortions beyond the twenty-eighth week of pregnancy were allowed, many medical practitioners—aware that advances in neo-natal medicine gave fetuses of between twenty-four and twenty-eight weeks' gestation a small chance of survival—refused to perform terminations beyond the twenty-fourth week.

In 1990, the Abortion Act was amended by the Human Fertilisation and Embryology Act. This act officially defined the upper limits for abortions at twenty-four weeks, though exceptions were permitted when the mother's life or health was in danger, or if there was a serious risk of severe fetal handicap. According to some experts, many doctors are so confused about the exception clause to the law that they are refusing to recommend abortion after twenty-four weeks, even when the fetus is afflicted by a lethal abnormality.

## Australia

Australian law is characteristically contradictory and confusing when it comes to the question of viability. Although only South Australia and the Northern Territory explicitly prohibit abortion beyond the twenty-eighth and the fourteenth week of pregnancy respectively (with exceptions in both cases for exceptional circumstances), recent studies have confirmed the difficulty all Australian women face in trying to obtain a termination beyond the twelfth or fourteenth week of pregnancy. For instance, despite the explicit legal limit of twenty-eight weeks in South Australia, only one service in the entire state currently provides abortions for women who are up to eighteen weeks pregnant.

The few Australian clinics that have cut-off dates later than fourteen weeks still tend to demand that women prove they are "deserving" before they will be "granted" an abortion, and refuse to perform post-twenty-week abortions in all cases. Clinics choose twenty weeks as their cut-off point because in 1978 the World Health Organization issued guidelines—now acknowledged to be based on political rather than medical considerations—that recommend against abortion beyond twenty weeks except in cases where the woman's life is in danger, or her fetus is severely deformed. Only the two clinics run by the medical director of Planned Parenthood of Australia, Dr. David Grundmann, will perform terminations beyond twenty weeks for "less critical" reasons. These reasons include situations where there are minor or possible fetal abnormalities, the woman has been raped, is an incest victim or is under the age of fifteen, the woman didn't know she was pregnant, has an intellectual impairment, or has experienced a catastrophic life-crisis such as the sudden death or desertion of a bread-winning partner.

that the development process is a continuum, with fertilization of the egg by the sperm at one end and birth at the other. Any attempt to place a wedge somewhere in this gradual process and declare that before the wedge the fetus doesn't matter, while after the wedge it does, is a decision that is as much a part of the sea of subjective values around abortion as any other.

•  •  •

A Wyoming woman is charged with child abuse for drinking when four months pregnant. Ultimately, the charges are dropped because the prosecutor could not prove injury to the fetus, which "was unavailable for examination."[6]

Once the fetus is understood to be a baby, pregnancy becomes merely an issue of fetal *location* and the woman merely the rather inconvenient "capsule" or "vessel" in which the fetus is held. The point of anti-choice propaganda and activism is to deny the importance of pregnancy in providing the necessary emotional and physical environment for the growth of the fetus and the development of the fetal–maternal relationship. In its place is substituted the image of a fully grown baby—a being no different from a new-born infant—trapped in the womb of its uncomprehending and potentially murderous mother. The commitment of the anti-choice movement to this view of pregnancy is demonstrated in its poster of a smiling baby. The caption reads: "Kill her now and it's called murder. Kill her three months ago and it's called abortion."

The now routine use of ultrasound in Western countries has been an important part of this shift. Ann Oakley has written about the ways in which ultrasound has changed the positions of the woman and the fetus relative to the doctor because its routine use

enables obstetricians to do without that classic piece of reproductive information—the date of the last menstrual period. Once it is believed that the machine is less fallible than the woman, then the woman does not need to be asked any more . . . This is in strong contrast to the message of the nineteenth-century textbooks which outlined a structure for the gynecological examination in which the doctor was at least as dependent on the patient's information as the patient was on the doctor's.[7]

Not only does ultrasound give doctors less reason to *speak* to women, it also gives them less reason to *look* at them. Bioethicist Barbara Rothman points out that during an ultrasound, the doctor must turn away from the pregnant woman in order to examine the fetus on the screen. Women gazing at the ultrasound image are also being directed for information about their pregnancy away from their bodies and their own experience. Of course, this understanding of the fetus as the primary patient in pregnancy and the woman as merely a "fetal container" is a result not just of the routine use of ultrasound, but of the increased usage of all of modern medicine's "fetal surveillance" techniques.[8] As the following quote (taken from an article about court-ordered cesareans) demonstrates, doctors are the first to admit that such techniques are fast becoming the mainstay of modern obstetric practice: "Advances in perinatology have emphasized electronic, ultrasonographic, and biochemical fetal surveillance techniques that identify the viable fetus as a patient for whom the obstetrician cares."[9]

When doctors see the fetus as their primary patient and the woman as either irrelevant or standing in the way of what they see as their job—ensuring that the fetus has all the medical interventions they perceive are in its interest—two things happen. The first is that pregnancy comes to be seen as an intrinsically conflictive relationship. Women's desires for themselves and their fetuses are deemed to conflict with what the "experts" believe are the fetuses' "best interests" (with the fetus falsely depicted here as a discrete and autonomous individual). The second thing that happens is that the use of brain-dead women's bodies to incubate non-viable fetuses appears not as the insane actions of a few fetally crazed medicos but the logical outcome of the shift from a woman-centered to a fetal-centered view of pregnancy.

•   •   •

A thirty-year-old woman suffered massive brain injuries after a motor vehicle accident. She was fifteen weeks pregnant. The woman was diagnosed as brain-dead on her tenth hospital day but supported with intensive care for 107 days after this diagnosis in order that she could continue gestating her fetus. A male infant was delivered after spontaneous labor began at thirty-two weeks' gestation, at which point the woman's life support machine was turned off. While she was on life support, she was treated for the standard complications of maintaining bodily functions after brain death. She developed diabetes, pituitary problems, and wide fluctuations in body temperature needing to be "controlled" by heating and cooling blankets. In addition, she developed and was treated for lung infections, was repeatedly transfused for "persistent" and "unexplained" anemia, and was administered CPR for one of two episodes of threatened heart failure. The treating doctors concluded that her case proved that "no clear lower limit exists that restricts the physician's ability to support the brain-dead pregnant patient."[10]

Commenting on a similar case, feminist bioethicist Laura Purdy notes that because "pregnant women are often still viewed primarily as mere fetal containers rather than as first-class citizens with their own pressing interests, dead pregnant women are . . . nearly as good as live ones."[11]

There are two clear and disturbing messages that get sent to all women when the "births" of children from the bodies of their long-dead mothers are announced in the media. The first is that who a pregnant woman is as a person, and a potential mother, is entirely separable from her body. The second is that the only thing a fetus really needs from its mother is her body, or more precisely her womb (given modern medicine's capacity to infuse or extract from the body in which the womb is situated all else necessary for fetal survival). In addition, such medical miracles implicitly ridicule pregnant women who so overrate their developing and anticipated relationship with their fetus and child-to-be that they name the fetus, as well as read and sing to it before it is born. Because, like fetuses, brain-dead women rarely ask questions or complain, they serve as an example to other women of the attributes most desired by doctors of their patients. Perhaps radical feminist Andrea Dworkin is not too far wrong when she concludes that in our patriarchal society, "the only good woman is a dead one."[12]

The depiction of pregnancy as a battle between mother and fetus ensures that all women—not just those who dare to question or disobey the doctors' orders—are seen to pose a significant health risk to their developing children. In the words of feminist bioethicist Christine Overall, "the pregnant woman cannot be trusted not to abuse [the foetus], pass on defective genes to it, or even kill it, let alone to protect it from environmental harm and give birth to it safely."[13]

• • •

In Washington, D.C. in 1987, twenty-seven-year-old Angela Carder, pregnant and dying of cancer, was forcibly strapped to an operating table and anesthetized so a team of doctors could operate to remove her twenty-five-week-old fetus from her body via cesarean section. The court order that allowed doctors to operate on Carder was issued after a hasty bedside courtroom was convened, complete with an advocate for Carder's fetus. Carder, who was both conscious and competent, had refused the operation upon the advice of her doctor, and with the support of her husband and family. As predicted, she and her fetus died shortly after they were separated. Three years later her family's appeal of the court order was upheld, although the dissenting judge supported the forced C section, citing as one of his reasons that Carder's fetus was a "captive" in her body.[14]

Angela Carder's story is by no means unique. Hundreds of women in the United States have either been ordered to undergo an intervention like a cesarean section or been physically detained because a doctor decides it is in the "best interests" of the fetus. Failing to follow the doctor's orders is no small offense in the United States. Two American teenaged mothers have been forced to "serve out" their pregnancies as hospital captives after doctors convinced the courts that the women's failure to properly manage their diabetes was endangering the health of their fetuses. Pamela Rae Stewart, a pregnant Californian woman, was jailed for fetal neglect after she ignored her doctor's advice to avoid sex and drugs and stay off her feet.[15]

• • •

In 1984 in Chicago, a Nigerian woman expecting triplets was hospitalized for the final period of her pregnancy. The woman and her husband steadfastly reiterated their unwillingness to consent to the cesarean section that doctors regarded as necessary for a safe multiple birth. As the woman's due date approached, doctors and hospital legal counsel obtained a court order granting the hospital administrator temporary custody of the triplets and authorizing a C section as soon as the woman went into labor. When she eventually did, her husband was forcibly removed from the hospital, the woman was strapped down, anaesthetized, and a C section was performed on her body. Several months later, her husband committed suicide.[16]

A recent study in the *New England Journal of Medicine* surveyed sixty-one American heads of fellowship programs and directors of divisions in maternal fetal medicine to find out where they stood on forced cesarean sections and other compulsory medical interventions in pregnancy. The results should send shivers up the spine of every woman considering pregnancy. A full 46 percent of these powerful (mostly) men thought that mothers who refused medical advice "deemed necessary for the fetus" should be detained in hospitals or other facilities so that "compliance" could be ensured. Approximately the same number thought that American courts should expand the range of conditions for which they could compel pregnant women to undergo medical interventions. Finally—this is the really scary one—26 percent advocated state surveillance of women in their third trimester who stay outside the hospital system. Twenty-two percent of this same group of medical practitioners went so far as to conclude that all home births should be illegal because they ". . . carried some inherent increase in risk and . . . every viable fetus ha[s] the right to live."[17]

Unfortunately, when it comes to issues of consent to medical treatment, the Australian medical profession is even more conservative than their American counterparts. In Australia, the "overwhelming tendency of the [Australian] courts to favor the opinion of doctors"[18] has led to a medical culture "antagonistic to many of the requirements for fostering and ensuring informed consent that have become part of routine medical . . . practice in the USA."[19] It is unlikely, therefore, that a similar survey of the attitudes of Australian doctors to forced medical treatment or detention of pregnant women would have any less worrying results.

In fact, the "doctor's orders" may soon include abortion, as well as unwanted cesareans and forced hospital detention; that is, if doctors like Margery Shaw have their way. Shaw believes that women should be required "to undergo genetic counselling before conception, to follow medically recommended regimens during pregnancy, to undergo fetal therapy to benefit 'the would-be child' and even to abort a fetus diagnosed as having a serious non-correctable defect."[20]

There is one critical assumption in every discussion of a woman's refusal of medical interventions: that the doctor knows best. The only way both the media and the medical profession get away with depicting women who refuse treatment as irrational, selfish, and unmotherly is the widely shared cultural assumption that there are *never* good reasons not to do what the doctor advises. But what if the doctor is wrong and the choices women make are *not* endangering their fetuses? What if what women are doing, or refusing to do, is actually in their fetuses' best interests?

Unsurprisingly, the belief that the doctor is always right and the patient always wrong has little in the way of facts to support it. In a study of women ordered by the courts to have cesarean sections, U.S. anthropologist Brigitte Jordan found that

some women were adamant that they didn't need a section. Some of these women had sections against their will, others had babies at home, or in hiding . . . [A]mong all the cases where a section occurred and in which an outcome assessment could be made, there was not a single one in which the section, in retrospect, appeared necessary.[21]

The majority of women forced to have cesareans, it is interesting to note, had already had at least one child. Jordan says that these findings started her thinking about "why and how it was the case that women's knowledge [about the need for a cesarean] didn't count, while medical knowledge carried the day. Which kind of knowledge was 'correct' obviously wasn't the decisive factor."[22]

Blind faith that the doctor knows best makes even less sense when we consider how enthusiastically the medical profession has supported numerous interventions in pregnancy that have later been shown to have caused serious harm to pregnant women and their children. In the 1960s, thousands of women took the drug DES (a synthetic estrogen prescribed to women to prevent miscarriage) on their doctor's advice, with what we now know are tragic—and multi-generational—consequences. Today, ultrasound is routinely used on pregnant women in the same way X-rays, now known to increase the risk of childhood cancer, were used on pregnant women from the 1920s to the 1950s. In 1994 in the Australian state of Victoria, fully 97 percent of women had at least one ultra-sound, and 43 percent had more than one.[23] This is despite the fact that a 1984 report by the joint National Institutes of Health/Food and Drug Administration Panel in the United States found "no clear benefit from routine use" and, more worryingly, no conclusive evidence of either its safety or harm.[25]

Finally, the scientific evidence upon which medical professionals often claim to make their decisions about what pregnant women should and should not do is often distorted. A 1989 study in *The Lancet* found that, while research findings "proving" that cocaine was connected with bad pregnancy outcomes were very likely to be accepted for presentation at the Society for Pediatric Research's annual meeting, studies that found no such connection had absolutely no chance of acceptance. Says award-winning American journalist Katha Pollitt:

While it's hard to imagine that anyone will ever show that heavy drug use or alcohol consumption is good for fetal development . . . when the dust settles (because the drug war is officially "won"? because someone finally looks at the newborns of Italy, where everyone drinks moderate amounts of wine with food, and finds them to be perfectly fine?) current scientific wisdom will look alarmist.[26]

• • •

A woman's offspring is her legacy to posterity, so it is common to assume that pregnancy is a cooperative enterprise between mother and child. But there is very little evidence for that. A lot of difficulties in pregnancy probably come about because there are genetic conflicts between what is best for the mother's genes and what is best for fetal genes.[27]

The anti-choice movement has lost little time in capitalizing on the legal and medical professions' view of pregnancy as a battlefield. The idea behind the now infamous anti-choice propaganda film *The Silent Scream* is that the fetus *consciously* struggles to survive an abortion. In the film, the audience becomes privy to what is purported to be an ultrasound image of an abortion of a twelve-week-old fetus (the fetus seen is actually a lot closer to twenty-four weeks' gestation). Narrated and interpreted by anti-choice activist Bernard Nathanson, the sped-up film footage purports to show the fetus "sensing mortal danger" and attempting to "escape" the suction cannula that has "invaded its sanctuary." At the conclusion of what we are told is the fetus's struggle with death, the fetus "rears back its head" in a "silent scream."

Celeste Condit explained why the film's viewers must be told what they are "seeing":

The ultrasound image [in the film] is so vague that without commentary many viewers would not have had the faintest idea what they were watching (as had been the case in my classes where I have shown students just the ultrasound image, without the sound or prior commentary). It is often very hard to see the fetus in this image. Moreover, even when the wispy "clouds on a radar screen" can be visualized as a fetus, the fetus does not appear as dramatically human. The resolution of the image is simply too poor to make a forceful argument in itself. The commentary . . . [is what] artfully tells the viewer what to see.[29]

Fetal researchers and abortion experts have repeatedly demonstrated the fraudulent nature of much of the film. Even the most radical fetal researchers rule out any possibility of the most primitive pain in the fetus prior to thirteen weeks' gestation, and screaming is impossible for lungs that have no air in them.[30] As Rosalind Petchesky points out, this literal kind of rebuttal, however, is "not very useful in helping us to understand the ideological power the film has despite its visual distortions and verbal fraud."[31] The film, in other words, is selling anti-choice "facts" about the fetus, "facts" that are meant to stir us up emotionally (the fetus wants to live! the fetus looks like a baby!) and lead us to make value judgments (the fetus *has a right* to life, the fetus *is* a person). However, even statements of fact possessing the usual characteristics associated with facts—some degree of validity—never lead incontrovertibly to statements of value. A similar point is made by Celeste Condit: "Without verbal commentary, pictures do not argue propositions. An image may suggest 'this looks like x,' but the assertion . . . that 'this is x,' must be verbally supplied. It is not surprising, therefore, that a great variety of commentary surround[s] the presentation of the images of the fetus."[32]

The anti-choice movement wants it both ways. On the one hand, films like *The Silent Scream* try to depict those who have abortions as callous women who have—for the sake of their own convenience—refused to accept their only legitimate role in life: motherhood. On the other hand, the anti-choice movement constantly challenges women's capacities to be moral mothers—to come up to scratch and meet "good mother" standards. The cases below are just a few examples of the second prong of this strategy.

• • •

> In 1987, an Illinois court allowed an infant to sue its mother for injuries suffered in an automobile accident when it was a five-month-old fetus. Five years later, a New Hampshire court came to a similar decision when it allowed a child born alive to sue its mother for injuries caused by negligence when she was seven months pregnant with that child: she was struck by a car. Her fetus, born by emergency cesarean section, suffered severe brain damage from the accident. The court agreed to hear the case on the grounds that the pregnant woman may have failed to act with the appropriate duty of care.[33]

The anti-choice strategy in seeking to prosecute women for "fetal abuse" is not only to establish the fetus as a person but to undermine all women's moral agency by establishing particular pregnant women to be indifferent and incompetent guardians of their fetuses' welfare. Once the pregnant woman's incompetence and indifference has been shown, the need for the anti-choice movement and the law to "protect" the fetus from its mother becomes clear.

Of course, pregnant women must be seen as less than moral agents, and incompetent decision makers, for the cesarean section forced upon the Nigerian woman carrying triplets to seem justified. Pregnancy must also be seen as an intrinsically adversarial relationship for it not to seem completely absurd that the hasty conference assembled beside Angela Carder's deathbed included someone representing and advocating for the fetus *other than* the fully conscious and competent Angela Carder.

Degrading women's competence and moral status works to validate the claims of the doctors, lawyers, judges and anti-choice representatives who claim to be spokespersons for the fetus. The need for a fetal spokesperson other than the woman is also reinforced by the media, which—having heard feminist organizations articulate the abortion "case" for women—feel the need to have a fetal "spokesperson" make the case for the fetus. It is worth noting that the distorted and self-serving view of pregnancy dished out by the anti-choice movement, which views pregnancy *not* as a special relationship between mother and fetus but as a battleground, could only have taken hold in a culture where women's points of view about pregnancy are largely absent. Iris Marion Young, a feminist scholar, notes dryly that the absence of knowledge about pregnancy from women's points of view, while regrettable, is not surprising. Says Young: "the specific experience of women has been absent from most of our culture's discourse about human experience and history."[34]

• • •

In South Australia, both first and second trimester abortions are performed in a hospital. In 1988, a situation of crisis developed around the provision of post-twelve-week abortions. A groundswell of discontent among medical staff surfaced, apparently catalyzed by the abortion, for social and economic reasons, of a twenty-four-week-old fetus. In other parts of the hospital, babies of around the same gestation were being saved. Nursing staff rebelled, refusing to participate in abortions when the pregnancy had progressed beyond twelve weeks. From 1988 until late 1990, South Australian women and girls more than three months pregnant travelled, at state government expense, to Melbourne or Sydney for abortions. The experience was traumatic for some. Those not prepared to go interstate continued the pregnancy.[35]

Feminists have long complained about the power—both in law and in practice—that the medical profession exercises over women's abortion decisions. While they argue that abortion is not a favor for the medical profession to bestow but an obligation for them to perform, many doctors, nurses, and medical institutions clearly think otherwise. One major concern highlighted by feminists has been the

## SECOND-TRIMESTER ABORTIONS

The vast majority of terminations take place well before the fetus is viable, or before week 24. In Australia, for example, 95 percent of abortions happen before week 14, with half of the remaining 5 percent performed before the eighteenth week. The vast majority of abortions performed after eighteen weeks are planned and wanted pregnancies that women choose to terminate because of "fatal or major fetal abnormalities or catastrophic changes in relationship, social or economic circumstances."[36] The balance are women who simply did not know they were pregnant. A gynecologist investigating the reasons why twelve British women needed late terminations found all

> had severe social and psychological problems. A twelve-year-old girl, for example, was found to be twenty-six weeks pregnant after her teacher noticed her stomach and sent her to a doctor. The girl's mother, whose husband was in prison, and who was preoccupied with other children, said she'd considered the weight gain to be "puppy fat." The girl said she had been raped in the lift of her block of flats. It later transpired that the alleged rapist was sexually involved with the mother.[37]

Women in Britain, Australia, and the United States have difficulty obtaining a second-trimester abortion, especially if they are poor or live in an area of the country where abortion attitudes are particularly conservative. One American study found that 22 percent of women on Medicaid having second-trimester abortions—Medicaid only funds abortions where the mother's life is at risk, or she is a victim of rape or incest—would have aborted in the first trimester if they could have found the necessary funds earlier. Another found almost half of the American women who have had abortions after fifteen weeks were delayed because of problems, usually financial, in arranging the abortion. Women also move from their first to their second trimester while waiting for publicly funded abortions in Britain and Australia. A recent Australian study found the following factors cause or contribute to delays that turn a first-trimester abortion into a later one: "limited provision of services, lengthy waiting periods for appointments, unhelpful or judgmental health professionals, failure to diagnose pregnancy and delayed or refused referral."[38]

high-handed and disrespectful way some practitioners deal with women's requests for abortion—a particular problem for British and Australian women because of the doctor's legally sanctioned role of gatekeeper. Vicki's story, told here, gives a good feel for this problem:

I'd asked to have my tubes tied, and they said yes, and put me on the waiting list. [When I found out I was pregnant] I went down there and said . . . "I am here to get a termination, when can it be done?" The doctor said "You can't have one, I won't do it" . . . and I said "Why won't you let me have it?" He said "Because you are 39, you are healthy, you are well, you have other children, there is nothing wrong with your pregnancy, there is nothing wrong with the other children you have and there is no reason why I would agree to that." I [was] . . . angry, furious, humiliated—that someone could put me down like that . . . It was humiliating, I ended up in tears and I am not normally that sort of person, I am usually a fairly aggressive person . . . He just humiliated me . . . I don't think that I have ever, in my life, felt like that.[39]

Sometimes doctors or entire hospitals simply refuse to provide abortion services. The problem is that while the law *permits* doctors to do abortions, it does not *require* them to do them. This is quite a different situation from that of compulsory education where the requirement that children be in school means that the State has a responsibility to provide adequate numbers of school places for all the children that need them. In Australia, hospitals and individual practitioners are allowed to provide as many publically funded abortions as necessary, or not to do any at all. Hospitals in the Australian Capital Territory, for example, will only do an abortion for a public patient if her life is at risk, or her fetus seriously deformed. In fact, the sum total of abortions performed by ACT hospitals every year is only two hundred. Until a freestanding abortion clinic opened a few years ago, the vast majority of women in the state were forced to travel—either to Melbourne or Sydney—for an abortion.

Periodically, the medical profession exercises its power by refusing, on grounds of conscience, to participate in existing abortion services. This is what happened in South Australia in 1988, when so many nurses refused to assist in second-trimester terminations that the service shut down altogether. While medical professionals stridently assert their rights to conscientiously object, it is clear that few of them understand the responsibilities that go along with this right. Even when essential services like abortion are *not* brought to a standstill, the right to conscientiously object is not unlimited, but must be balanced against the rights of patients to health care and the consequences to them of not getting this care. However, once the actions of medical professionals actually shut down a service, the conscientious objections of health care providers can never be justified. They have simply put their patients at too great a risk.

But even if some medicos believe their rights to autonomy (the basis of the right to conscientiously object) are so important that they justify putting patients at risk, they need to understand that once their refusal to provide care has led to a shutdown of an essential medical service, they aren't acting as conscientious objectors any more. Instead, their actions have become political ones—acts of civil disobedience—and they have become civil dissenters. A civil dissenter has a number of obligations to the community, the most important of which is to expect and accept arrest and punishment for having failed to fulfill obligations. This is precisely the attitude of those who refused to serve in Vietnam, and many of these young men did, in fact, go to jail. Other consequences that may befall civil dissenters are dismissal from their jobs, or hefty fines.[40]

The bottom line, in other words, is that medical professionals should put their money where their anti-choice mouths are. If their ethical opposition to abortion is sincere, they should be willing to pay the price for exercising their autonomy at the cost of the autonomy of their patients. If they are not acting from their most fundamental moral convictions, they should ensure that they do not disregard their obligations to patient care so lightly.

I say all this because evidence suggests that it is not the fundamental moral questions about abortion that really concern doctors and nurses, but the practical, work-related issues about who gets stuck doing how many of the "dirty" jobs. According to a South Australian clinical nurse, Di Krutli, concerns about nurses getting stuck with caring for second-trimester abortion patients seem to be the crux of many of the South Australian nurses' conscientious objections to abortion:

The procedure for a mid-trimester termination was either a saline or pros-
taglandin injected [into the woman's womb] to induce labor. The women
actually delivered (or aborted) on the ward, either in bed or in a bedpan.
The nurse was left with all the difficult work—you could actually say all
the "dirty" work . . . [T]he nurse had to weigh the fetus, the nurse had to
place the fetus in a bag and transport it to a mortuary, the nurse had to
clean bed, patients, and any remaining products. The nurse had to answer
patients' questions, sometimes distressing, about the size, appearance, sex,
disposal of the fetus and whether it was still alive. The nurse had to deal
with distressed patients and relatives . . .[41]

There are clearly a large number of things medical professionals
get stuck with doing that they'd rather not do (although it's likely
that the nursing profession gets stuck with a disproportionate number of them): cleaning up vomit, telling patients they've got cancer,
delivering a baby with gross birth defects. It's unlikely many people
would feel it fair for medical professionals to "conscientiously object" their way out of doing these tasks. The reality is they simply
have to be done, and it's part of the medical professionals' job to do
them. Don't like it, we'd think, then get another job. Abortion provision, too, is simply part of the obligation to patient care that the
medical professional signs on to when they take the job. Certainly
this attitude is the one taken by American obstetrician David
Grimes: "My feelings as a doctor should never interfere with what I
do for my patients. There are many aspects of medicine that may
not be particularly fun or enjoyable or pleasant, but I have an ethical obligation to do what's best for my patients and not take my
own personal convenience into consideration."[42]

That said, there is little doubt that a second-trimester "labor and
birth" abortion is a difficult and traumatic procedure, certainly for
the attending nurse but mostly for the pain-racked and often griev-
ing mother who must give birth to a dead baby. The irony is that the
reason Australian nurses have to do the "dirty work" of caring for
women having second-trimester instillation abortions is because
Australian doctors continue to refuse to perform the second-
trimester procedure, dilatation and evacuation, which has been
medically proven to be in the best interests of the pregnant woman
(it's been the method of choice in the United States for years). The
recent NHMRC report into abortion found that the Australian

medical profession continues to force women to abort later pregnancies by "giving birth"—even women terminating intended pregnancies because of severe fetal defects—despite the increased dangers and difficulties of this method for both women and nursing staff:

Instillation methods have a higher mortality than Dilatation and Evacuation and similar to childbirth itself. In those States of Australia where they are still routinely used, instillation methods appear to be favored by doctors but not by patients or support staff. In the USA, Dilatation and Evacuation has been the recommended method from 13 to 16 weeks since 1978 but Dilatation and breech eXtraction (D and X) is emerging as the favored method, especially after 16 weeks. Although very taxing on the provider, it is preferred by other staff and the woman. There is a very low complication rate in skilled hands.[43]

For many women, however, the pain of a second-trimester labor abortion is preferable to that of raising a severely or fatally handicapped child. In recent years, there has been greater recognition of the impact on families of caring for a severely disabled child. In their controversial book *Should the Baby Live?*, bioethicists Peter Singer and Helga Kuhse cite an article written by an anonymous Melbourne woman whose sister, Barbara, had been born with brain damage caused by rubella. The woman wrote the letter in response to what she felt were the glib statements about the "rights of the child" made by someone on a talk-back radio program about severely disabled infants.

Barbara did not walk until she was four, was not toilet trained until she was seven, had frequent fits, and slept only two hours a day. Her parents quarreled violently, with one repeatedly threatening to leave. The woman wrote that she would vomit each night on her way home from school because she was so frightened of what she might find at home. She concluded:

And through it all Barbara continued to move like a demented destroyer, hyped up by the constant adrenaline that drowned all calm and logic, unmoved by my father kicking and bellowing at my brother, lashing out at him constantly with the strap, she babbled on and on, shaking you and demanding a response, rocking in her chair and making wild noises, or moving about shifting things and throwing tantrums at every frustration. And never sleeping.[44]

That women are being forced to bear a severely handicapped

child against their will is yet another tragedy of the obsession with fetal viability.

• • •

In 1987 in the United Kingdom, a Mrs. Rance learned that her twenty-seven-week-old fetus had severe spina bifida—a condition that results in paralysis, incontinence, and in some cases mental retardation. She approached the National Health Service for an abortion but was refused on the grounds that the child was viable—capable of being born alive. She sued and lost, and was forced to have the child, which was born—as expected—severely disabled.[45]

What the decision in the Rance case made clear was that the twenty-eight-week legislative limit in Britain on abortions was entirely vulnerable to changes in technology. Viability, in other words, was not a fixed point, but one that could go as low as technological change would permit. Future Mrs. Rances may need to abort their severely damaged fetuses prior to the twentieth week of pregnancy, or perhaps even the eighteenth. In order for this to happen, fetal diagnostic techniques will also have to change with the times. The results of the most common and low-risk technique—amniocentesis—are typically unavailable before the eighteenth week of pregnancy, sometimes not earlier than the twentieth or twenty-second week.

In Britain, the Rance case coincided with attempts by anti-choice politicians to use the viability issue to curtail British women's access to second-trimester abortions. Several parliamentarians had attempted to pass bills that sought to reduce the time in which women could choose abortion to twenty weeks in one instance, eighteen in the other. Neither piece of legislation was passed. However, the dual pressures of the Rance judgment, and pressure for legislative change from anti-choice politicians, finally forced the amendment of the 1967 Abortion Act by the Human Fertilization and Embryology Act (HFEA), 1990. The HFEA subtracts four weeks from the period in which women may legally obtain an abortion by moving the legal limit from twenty-eight to twenty-four weeks.

In fact, the vast majority of British doctors had been refusing to perform post-twenty-four-week abortions for years. In 1992, in the United Kingdom, there were only sixty-three of these abortions performed, and almost every one of these cases involved a seriously abnormal fetus. Janet Hadley believes that many doctors have stopped doing second-trimester terminations altogether—even for lethal abnormalities—because they find the exception clause of the new law, which permits them to perform abortions after the twenty-fourth week if the fetus is severely handicapped, confusing.

● ● ●

You are two months pregnant. You cannot raise the child and so must decide between having an abortion or carrying the child to term and giving it up for adoption. As you consider these options, a doctor approaches and informs you about a wonderful new option. Thanks to technology, it is now possible for you to abort your fetus without killing it. Your fetus can be extracted from your body and transferred to an artificial womb, where it will be grown for nine months and then put up for adoption. "Are you interested?" he asks.

This is the scenario I put to the women I interviewed for my research. In essence, I was asking women to respond to the Singer and Wells proposal for abortions of the future. It is the only nightmare scenario raised in this chapter so far that remains—at least for the time being—safely in the future. But how safely? While it may be a matter of debate how many years before we reach the point where fetuses as young as eight or twelve weeks could survive in neo-natal intensive-care wards, many medical professionals have little doubt that the futuristic world envisioned by Singer and Wells will one day come to pass. The approach of medical scientists to ectogenesis is being made along several different paths.

Scientists have gained knowledge about ectogenesis as a by-product of the extensive work being done in the area of infertility treatments like in-vitro fertilization (IVF). IVF success rates are known to be as low as eight pregnancies for every one hundred women completing a single treatment.[46] Since 1978, when the first test-tube baby was born, infertility specialists have been desperately trying to improve these statistics. Women leave IVF programs for numerous reasons, among them the painful and humiliating nature of many procedures with benign names like "egg retrieval" and "embryo transfer." Another reason women quit is the failure of their eggs and the sperm to join together and form a viable embryo. Viable embryos must get high grades in a number of areas: their appearance and clarity, the tightness of the cell constellation, and the rate of cell growth. While IVF practitioners often blame women for treatment failures, telling them their eggs are "too old" or just not "good enough," behind the scenes they have been searching for ways to improve egg viability by improving the culture liquid in which sperm and eggs fertilize and divide.[47] The search for better culture fluid is done via experimentation on human and mouse embryos. Recently, an Australian IVF team predicted an up-turn in their "take-home baby rate" with increased use of both a new culture fluid "recipe" and a technique for assessing the health of the embryos so only the healthiest ones were transferred to the woman.[48] New culture fluids were also responsible for the recent "success" of one Melbourne IVF team in extending the growth period of embryos in petri dishes from three to five days. The IVF team boasted that the 40 percent success rate achieved with this method is better than the 30 percent rate of natural conception.[49]

This same group of doctors is also freezing human ovaries. When a woman wishes to conceive, her ovaries will either be reimplanted or the eggs contained within them will be "harvested" for in vitro fertilization. Ovary freezing has already been successful in tests using pieces of ovary from sheep and mice. While the technique will initially only be offered to women who have lost their ovaries due to cancer, endometriosis, or premature menopause, it may one day be made available to any woman who wants to preserve her fertility for the future.[50]

The use of donor eggs in the IVF program has taught scientists another lesson essential to the ultimate success of the ectogenetic womb—that a fetus need not grow in the uterus of its genetic mother to survive. Countless babies have now been conceived in the United States, Britain, and Australia from donor eggs. The women who bear these children are their gestational, but not genetic, mothers. Brain-dead women have also taught scientists pursuing ectogenesis a valuable lesson. Because these women's pregnancies can be preserved by hooking their bodies up to life-support machines (one brain-dead woman actually conceived a child after her body was raped), it seems possible that machines may be just as good as live women at "conceiving" and "giving birth" to children.

The steady lowering of the age of fetal viability also takes us closer and closer to the Singer and Wells abortion solution. With fetuses as young as twenty-two weeks being "salvaged" in the neonatal wards of many Western nations, some neonatologists have suggested that over the next few decades it will become possible to save the lives of babies born after only sixteen to eighteen weeks in the maternal womb.[51]

Perhaps it may—as Singer and Wells suggest—become possible for technology to advance so far that we are able to rescue first-trimester fetuses. This would mean that the roughly 95 percent of abortions that now take place in the first trimester could become fetal *evacuations*. The fetus would be removed alive from its mother's body and placed in an ectogenetic womb capable of sustaining its life. When fully mature, it would be put up for adoption.

Some scientists are directly investigating the possibility of a successful full- or part-term ectogenetic pregnancy. In 1988, a group of Italian scientists pieced together a contraption made of the extracted uteri of women with cancer.[52] They were able to keep an embryo alive in this artificial womb for over fifty-two hours. Their goal? To gain the knowledge necessary to take total ectogenesis—the gestation of a human from an embryo to a nine-month-old baby in an artificial womb—from the realms of science fiction to reality. More recently, Japanese scientists incubated a partially developed goat kid from 120 days (the equivalent of the twentieth to twenty-fourth gestational week of a human fetus) until it was ready to be born, seventeen days later.[53] Despite obvious developmental problems with the resulting kid—it was unable to stand or breathe by itself—the scientists were pleased with the results, making it likely they'll continue their work in the future.

• • •

Far from being the kooky prediction of a couple of out-of-touch academics, the Singer–Wells solution is simply the logical outcome of the way we have come to see fetuses, women, and pregnancy. For it to actually come to pass, two conditions must be met. First, technology must advance to the point where it is medically possible to keep a woman's first-trimester fetus alive in an artificial womb. Second, we must look at pregnancy as nothing but an issue of fetal location, and the pregnant relationship as an inherently adversarial one. We must also view the termination of pregnancy and the death of the fetus as entirely separate events.

We're already halfway there.

# · 4 ·

# Pregnancy

It is impossible to understand women's moral stance on abortion without understanding how they think about and experience pregnancy. Yet pregnancy is rarely discussed when the ethics of abortion are being considered, and pregnant women are rarely mentioned or pictured in anti-choice materials. One reason for this is that most anti-choice material and most academic ethicists have focused exclusively on whether abortion—the abstract act of terminating a pregnancy—is right or wrong. In these discussions, the conversation *starts* at the point at which a woman is deciding the fate of her unplanned pregnancy, with all that has come prior to this decision (and puts the decision in context) entirely ignored. Alternately, ethicists and anti-choice activists have viewed pregnancy as the "bed" women must lie in if they have been "irresponsible" with contraception.

My research shows that women's abortion ethics focus precisely on what ethicists and the anti-choice movement ignore—the particular abortions of particular women. To have an opinion about the ethics of a particular abortion and a particular aborting woman, the women in my study needed to know the aborting woman's attitude not just to the abortion, but to pregnancy and to motherhood. They wanted to feel comfortable not only with the circumstances surrounding her pregnancy, but with the meaning—in a holistic sense—the woman makes of her pregnancy.

## Genetics or Gestation

The other reason why ethicists ignore or underplay the importance of women's experiences and understandings of pregnancy is that the relationship pregnancy establishes between women and their fetuses and the children they become is something only women experience. It is not hard to imagine why, in a world dominated by the views of men, the importance of a genetic, rather than a gestational, connection to one's children has paramount importance. The British Warnock Report on reproductive technologies, for example, focused on the rights of genetic parents over children and the rights of children to know and inherit from their genetic forebears. The grounding belief of Australian social policy until the late 1960s was that the connection between mother and child didn't matter. This was the basis for brutal policies like the forced removal of Aboriginal children from their biological mothers and the coercion of unwed women to relinquish their babies for adoption. But the view that it is genetics, not gestation, that matters is slowly being challenged. For instance, a recent study reported in the *Journal of Medical Ethics* found more women would prefer to be birth mothers than genetic mothers.[1] Regis Dunne argues that: "Biological relationships are real, part of nature, flesh, blood and human existence. They persist as long as life itself, and though they may be complemented by social relationships, they cannot be supplanted, nor can they be negated by legal fiction, nor by persuasive twists of language."[2]

Jungian psychiatrist and feminist Dr. Naomi Lowinsky believes that the fact of women's and men's differing contributions to bearing children means the connections they have with those children are qualitatively different:

Patriarchal lineage is . . . abstract . . . It is about the handing down of names . . . legitimacy, inheritance, marriage contracts . . . The distinction is tied to the difference in the experience of female conceiving and male begetting. No woman has to wonder whether it is her child she is bearing; she has conceived the child. She has carnal self knowledge of her maternity as the baby develops within her. But a man, leaving his seed in the darkness of a woman, has to [act so as to] assure himself of his claim to the future.[3]

Famous anthropologist Margaret Mead pointed out years ago that male-dominated civilizations have consistently struggled to "define the male role [in procreation] satisfactorily enough for men."[4] Similarly, philosopher Mary O'Brien believes that what Freud's female followers have called "womb envy" is the basis of the relentless desire of male-dominated cultures to create institutions that ". . . will not only subdue the waywardness of women but also give men an illusion of procreative continuity and power."[5]

It appears, however, that the nearly universal concerns men have about paternity may be justified. A recent study in a small English town found that fully 30 percent of husbands could not actually have fathered "their" children.

Elizabeth Kane, the first "surrogate" mother, says she believed the male fiction that "the only issue of importance is where the egg or the sperm originates."[7] She had to learn the hard way about the special and unbreakable bond that develops between women and their children during pregnancy. Kane recalled lying on the delivery table, with the couple who'd commissioned her to bear a child for them holding her newborn son in their arms:

At that moment, I thought it would not matter to me if I never saw him again . . . It had not once entered my mind that, even though the doctor had physically disconnected us in cutting the umbilical cord, I would be attached to this child by a heartstring for the rest of my life. I know now that our judicial system might be able to take a baby from a woman's arms, but it can never remove that child from her heart or memory.[8]

## Pregnancy: Myths and Facts

An amazing assortment of myths and assumptions surround pregnancy. They include the belief that all unplanned pregnancies are due to improper or non-use of "reliable" contraceptive measures; all unplanned pregnancies are unwanted; all unwanted pregnancies end in abortion; and women who have unplanned pregnancies are teenagers, promiscuous, ignorant of both the facts of life and the miracles of modern contraception, and/or are women who either can't afford or are unable to get their hands on reliable birth control methods. It is assumed that all women would rather prevent pregnancy than interrupt it, that birth control is a woman's responsibility, and that unplanned pregnancy is a woman's fault.

The facts, as usual, tell a different story. For starters, while half of the world's pregnancies are unplanned, only half of those are unwanted. As already mentioned, the number of unplanned pregnancies in Europe and Australia is even higher—two out of three. But of the Australian pregnancies that were unwanted, less than half ended in abortion. Most abortions are had by unmarried women in their early twenties, though married women account for approximately one-quarter of those having abortions in Australia and 18 percent of those having abortions in the United States. One in three Australian women will have an abortion before the sunset of her reproductive years.[9]

## The Myth of Controllable Fertility

One of the most popular and dangerous myths perpetrated in the twentieth century is that women's fertility is entirely controllable using modern methods. Ha! In fact, the number of women who will become pregnant within a year using many modern contraceptive methods is jaw-droppingly high. Over the course of a year, 36 percent of women will become pregnant if they use the cervical cap or sponge, 18 percent if they use the diaphragm, 3 percent if they use the pill, and 12 percent if their partners use a condom.[10] One American study found that condom failure was responsible for 32 percent of the pregnancies in women seeking abortions.[11] The IUD is nothing to write home about either, with two of forty women in one study becoming pregnant with one inserted.[12] A counselor at an American abortion clinic put it this way: "The number of IUDs that are still in place before we do a suction abortion is just amazing. Every time I see that, I go home and sleep in the guest room for a week."[13]

In addition, many doctors seem to be making a habit of (mistakenly) telling women and men that they are likely to be infertile for one reason or another. In her book on contraceptive risk-taking, Kristin Luker notes that fully two-thirds of the pregnant women she interviewed had been told by their gynecologists that they would have trouble conceiving. In fact, much of what modern medicine currently terms infertility may turn out to be an artifact of modern medical definitions. Nowadays, a couple is stamped "infertile" by the medical profession—particularly those in the IVF industry—

after one year of unprotected intercourse without conception. This is despite the fact that several studies have shown that the majority of the approximately 20 percent of couples who take longer than a year to conceive will eventually become pregnant without any medical intervention at all.[14] It is also a sad fact that some of the women and men who really are infertile are the product of the unabashed experimentation by the medical profession on their mothers. Some of the women and men queuing for expensive infertility treatment today, for instance, were born in the 1960s of mothers who'd been prescribed DES. DES is now recognized as the cause of genital abnormalities and cancer in the daughters and sons of the women who took it. What's even more frightening is that some of the more popular drugs given to women on IVF programs today are under suspicion of causing defects in the reproductive systems of this new generation of children. Amazingly, the medical profession has decided—because of the absence of definitive proof—to keep giving women the suspect drugs until a statistically significant number of their daughters and sons have reached adolescence and can examined for defects and disease.[15]

It is a myth that the pill and the IUD—promoted as the only substantially user-controlled and reliable methods of avoiding pregnancy—are without significant side-effects. Of the 85 percent of Australian women who use either, many complain that the IUD makes them feel physically uncomfortable and the pill leaves them feeling plain unwell. Moreover, women have begun to be suspicious of medical assurance that these methods are totally safe. Hard to blame them. Until Barbara Seaman's book *The Doctor's Case Against the Pill* was published in 1969—linking the pill to increased risks of thrombosis and certain forms of cancer—the medical profession refused to acknowledge there were *any* risks associated with the pill. Little has changed. Until October 1994, it would have been next to impossible to find a medical professional who wouldn't have affirmed the new generation of oral contraceptives as being "extremely safe." Now, the still unanswered questions about the elevated risk of blood clots run by women taking these pills has led the British government to warn women not to take them at all, and German authorities to suggest that certain groups of women avoid them.[16] In the same way, the Dalkon Shield IUD was promoted as the "perfect alternative" to the pill until seventeen women died from using it, and countless others found themselves with infections that caused septic abortions and/or infertility.[17]

In a recent foray to Family Planning Australia, I was strongly urged to "get on the pill." I explained to my counselor that the pill made me sick, and the mini-pill gave me migraines. When she suggested the IUD, I said that the Dalkon Shield fiasco and the bad experiences of several of my friends—one bled so much she was calling in sick to work one day a month and the other had to have minor surgery when it disappeared, string and all, into her uterus— made me wary.

"They do say the new ones don't have whatever caused the problems with the Dalkon Shield," she'd ventured.

"But I don't trust *them*," I'd said.

"Fair enough too," she'd conceded, trotting off to get me a tube of cream for my cap.

## The Myth about Risk-taking

The most pernicious myths about pregnancy come from sexist assumptions and expectations about women's attitudes to and behavior around sex, marriage, and motherhood.

The first myth is that people—and women are included here— judge the risks of a particular situation in the same way that statisticians do. Pregnancy is a great example of how this is simply not the case. According to the stats, roughly 80 percent of women not practicing contraception will eventually become pregnant. But Kristin Luker found in her research on women's contraceptive decisions that many women did not necessarily see the odds in the same way:

[women] are usually aware of the odds of pregnancy . . . but for them individually the chances are zero or one: either they get pregnant or they do not. One simply cannot translate an 80 percent chance of pregnancy *over the long run* into being 80 percent pregnant, so the risk-taking is very different for them than for statisticians.[18]

Many women simply deny the possibility of pregnancy. According to West Australian family planning counselor Antonia Clissa, the most often repeated statement made in counselling sessions is, "I never thought it would happen to me."

There are a wide range of practices in every society that everyone says they disapprove of, but do anyway. According to Luker, contraception is one such practice where there is "widespread private deviance from official norms, but general public support of them."[19] In reality, people—and again women are included here—take risks. They smoke cigarettes, climb mountains, bungee jump, and drive without seat belts. The experts believe such risk-taking is normal: "most well-adjusted individuals habitually take chances with their health and safety, and . . . most persons take some risks in their lives eventually."[20]

When women take risks with contraception, however, the same experts deem them "neurotic, deviant and unrealistic."[21] Becoming pregnant when one does not wish to become a mother is, according to one commentator, evidence of a woman's "distorted and unrealistic way out of inner difficulties and is thus comparable to neurotic symptoms on the one hand and delinquent behavior on the other." According to another, unwanted pregnancy indicates a personality that is both "immature" and "pathological."[22]

It is estimated that the average woman would have over ten abortions during her reproductive lifetime if no other forms of birth control were available. What this means is that a woman not practicing contraception may have a large number of sexual encounters that *do not* result in pregnancy, until the one that finally does. One twenty-eight-year-old woman interviewed by Linda Francke recounted how she lived with her eighteen-year-old lover for two years, having "constant" sex, before finally falling pregnant. Often, the failure to fall pregnant is not seen as a lucky triumph over the inevitable odds, but proof to the woman that she or her partner is not fertile.

Among the number of (almost always unconscious) reasons women have for becoming pregnant is to confirm their fertility. While school sex education was all about convincing girls that even looking at a boy while naked would make them pregnant, recent press about infertility makes women fear that, no matter how hard they try, they may never get pregnant. The result is that many women over the age of twenty-five are convinced they're infertile if they have never been pregnant. In fact, and this is no exaggeration, every mother I know, bar one, was convinced she was infertile prior to conceiving her first child. The exception? A woman who'd previously had an abortion. Interestingly, many of these women had chosen to take the pill because it offered such good protection against pregnancy, and had then begun to fear—along with some members of the medical profession—that prolonged pill use could damage their fertility. Because most women ultimately do want to have kids, widespread panic about the "infertility epidemic" tends to push many women to subconsciously "test" that their apparatus is in working order.

In addition to demonstrating fertility, pregnancy may offer a woman other benefits. Again, however, Kristin Luker reminds us that women's cost/benefit calculations differ from the experts':

The woman must perceive contraception as costly before risk-taking can occur; but the benefits of pregnancy never become actual until at least a month after the decision to take a risk has been made. In other words, the decision to take a contraceptive risk is typically based on the *immediate* costs of contraception and the *anticipated* benefits of pregnancy. The difference is important, because for the women . . . [I studied] the potential benefits of pregnancy seldom became real: they vanished with the verdict of a positive pregnancy test or were later outweighed by the actual costs of the pregnancy . . . Therefore what we are examining are . . . the benefits anticipated at the time of the decision to take a contraceptive risk.[23]

Many of the women in Luker's study felt pregnancy would earn them the stamp of approval from their parents, friends, and society at large because pregnancy would "prove" their womanhood and their value as potential mothers. Some women used pregnancy as a plea for support either from their parents or from "experts" in the helping professions.

## Responsibility and the Sexual Double Standard

The sexual double standard ensures that even though it takes both sexes to make a pregnancy, when one happens, it is then largely seen as the woman's fault. In large part, this is a result of the Western approach to family planning research and education, which is almost solely focused on controlling the reproductive systems of women. According to Dr. David Handelsman, director of the Andrology Unit at the Royal Prince Alfred Hospital in Sydney, it is the "low priority accorded to male contraceptive development and the consequent lack of resources for research and development in male reproductive medicine" that is responsible for the lack of a hormonal contraceptive alternative for men.[24] Family planning expert and feminist Judith Bruce says that when it comes to contraceptive education, things are no better: "conventional approaches to fertility reduction have been characterised by an over-reliance on "men's behaviour [and] neglect of male sexual and contraceptive behaviour."[25]

Sadly, women have bought into the sexual double standard about responsibility for pregnancy. For instance, while women are nearly twice as likely as men to use contraception, if they do become pregnant, they almost always shoulder the blame. One woman remembers when she was first told she was pregnant: "my whole face turned red . . . I just felt real stupid . . . I kind of felt like it was all my fault and that was a big burden."[26] Another said: "I know it took two of us to get pregnant but I still feel I shouldn't have let it happen. After all, I'm the one that's pregnant. It's my fault!"[27]

Not only do women believe themselves solely responsible, and judge themselves harshly when they become pregnant, they fear others will do the same. Modern women, according to one of the women I interviewed, are not supposed to "lose control" of their bodies:

CHARITY: There's more and more pressure to plan. To be completely in control of your body, so if you fall pregnant, you've done it deliberately, and you know when you're going to fall pregnant. Organization . . . Because women are expected to do more and more things in their lives and to have a spot worked in to have children.

LC: So if you get pregnant and it isn't planned, you've made an error and people will blame you for it?

CHARITY: Yeah.

A great many men, on the other hand, have no scruples when it comes to contraception. Forget about initiating discussions about contraception in their relationships, or actually going themselves to the drug store to purchase a packet of condoms, research suggests many men will go to amazing lengths to avoid wearing the condoms women provide for them even when they know she is extremely concerned about becoming pregnant. In order to "get out" of wearing condoms, men have told some amazing lies. In the 1970s, Francke told of the bewilderment of one pregnant woman who'd been told by her boyfriend he'd had a vasectomy, and been shown the scar to prove it. When asked by abortion clinic staff where the scar was, the woman had lifted up her arm and pointed to her armpit. Another woman was so nervous about becoming pregnant she would break out in hives every time her boyfriend entered the room. She said that while he'd once bought a condom "he . . . didn't like it" and had taken it "right off."[29]

In the 1990s, little has changed regarding men's aversion to condoms, despite the promotion of condoms as a necessary part of sex in the era of AIDS. Some men describe using them as the equivalent of taking a shower with a raincoat on, and refuse to wear them. And for their part, the majority of women still fail to insist that—as one Australian promotional campaign put it—"if it's not on, it's not on." In the words of one Australian AIDS educator: "Condoms have been focussed on as our best line of defense against AIDS and other RDs, but appear to still be shunned and relegated to being used inconsistently or not at all."[30]

Sadly, even married men with "liberated views" have little interest in sharing the responsibility for contraception. American researchers looking at the connections between men's attitudes to sex roles and their contraceptive behavior have recently concluded that "Egalitarian sex-role preferences do not necessarily translate into a strong commitment to share contraceptive responsibility."[31]

What is really depressing, however, are the reasons many women give for not insisting their sexual partners wear condoms. Because having a condom is evidence a girl is both planning and prepared for sex, it seems many men (and some women) are convinced that women who do carry them are "easy" or "sluts." One young Australian woman put it this way: "If I've got a condom in my bag he thinks I'm ready [for sex]: she's done it before, she must sleep around. It's better it happens naturally, spontaneously, then there's no blame."[32]

While for a woman in the 1970s the dilemma was between protecting her reputation as a "nice girl" and protecting herself against an unplanned pregnancy, today's woman needs to balance her "reputation" against the need to avoid not only pregnancy but sexually transmitted diseases that kill. It is frightening to think how many people—women and men—will contract the AIDS virus because social attitudes haven't changed half as quickly as the diseases that exploit them.

## Women's Experience of Pregnancy

Most non-Western societies see the first-time pregnant woman as both vulnerable and powerful because she is in transition from the role and status of child to that of mother. Having left one identity but not yet entered another, she is seen as "liminal," posing a danger to those around her, especially men. In some agricultural communities, pregnant women are believed to have the power to spoil food, sour milk, and still the growth of plants.[33]

Western cultures have tended to distort ancient views about pregnant women's liminal status in two ways. First, instead of viewing women as threats to their communities or to men, in Western cultures the woman is seen as a danger to her fetus. Second, instead of viewing pregnancy as a natural part of the reproductive lives of healthy women, Western cultures see pregnancy as an illness. The most popular pregnancy manuals tell pregnant women, both by what is included and by what is omitted, that the only issue of valid concern for a pregnant woman is her fetus's—and by extension her own—health. The introduction to the wildly popular *What to Expect When You're Expecting* notes that:

According to the media, threats to the pregnant lurked everywhere: in the air we breathed, in the food we ate, in the water we drank, at the dentist's office, in the drugstore, even at home. My doctor offered some solace, of course, but only when I was able to summon up the courage to phone . . .

Was I . . . alone in my fears? Far from it. Worry, according to one study, is one of the most common complaints of pregnancy . . . but though a little worry is normal . . . a lot of worry is an unnecessary waste of what should be a blissfully happy time. Despite all that we hear, read and worry about, never before in the history of reproduction has it been safer to have a baby.[34]

When pregnancy is turned from a ritual state into an illness, pregnant women are no longer viewed as powerful creators, but as patients. According to Sheila Kitzinger, the job of the pregnant patient in a modern Western hospital is to "hand herself over to its care without asking too many questions or disrupting the smooth running of the institution. Any woman who [is] hoping for negotiation and discussion with her care-givers is likely to be frustrated the very first time she attends an antenatal clinic."[35]

Because pregnancy is seen as an illness, researchers have approached it strictly from a medical perspective. For example, a recent study of Australian women's experiences of motherhood restricted its considerations of pregnancy to the evaluations women gave of their antenatal care.[36] With few exceptions, women's experience of pregnancy and birth has been of little interest to anyone besides "anthropologists concerned with childbirth in cultures other than their own."[37]

For most women, however, pregnancy is experienced as much more than a medical event. Looking back on her pregnancy, one woman remembers: "I felt at the same time more vulnerable and more powerful than ever."[38] A feminist academic described her experience of pregnancy this way:

The integrity of my body is undermined in pregnancy . . . by the fact that the boundaries of my body are . . . in flux. In pregnancy I literally do not have a firm sense of where my body ends, and the world begins. My automatic body habits become dislodged, the continuity between my customary body and my body at this moment is broken.[39]

One reason so little has been written about women's experience of pregnancy is that it is difficult to find words and concepts that do it justice in our "man-made" language.[40] When Iris Young went to the library in search of information on women's experience of pregnancy, she found:

The library card catalogue contains dozens of entries under the heading "pregnancy": clinical treatises detailing signs of morbidity; volumes cataloguing studies of fetal development, with elaborate drawings; or popular manuals in which physicians and others give advice on diet and exercise for the pregnant woman. It is either a state of the developing foetus, for which the woman is container; or it is an objective, observable process coming under scientific scrutiny; or it becomes objectified by the woman herself, as a "condition" in which she must "take care of herself." Except perhaps for one insignificant diary, no card appears listing a work which, as [French philosopher Julia] Kristeva puts it, is "concerned with the subject, the mother as the site of her own proceedings."[41]

But it has not just been patriarchal culture that has sidelined motherhood. Until the early 1980s, the second wave of white middle-class feminists also studiously avoided both topics, convinced pregnancy and motherhood were the sources of women's oppression. One feminist academic, Rivka Polantrick, recalled that:

As a young woman in the late 1960s, I had internalized an attitude from my radical feminist circles that becoming a mother meant getting mired in women's oppression. By the early 1980s, I had experienced a trend in White feminism toward revaluing motherhood, but I still associated it with being confined, curtailed, and diminished.[42]

Similarly, an editor of a recent anthology of fiction about motherhood remembered that she too

didn't want to be pregnant. Or so I thought, through my vehement twenties and well into my still-strident thirties. I was a seventies feminist for whom a woman's creative freedom meant a room of one's own, and no one to answer to whenever I felt like taking in a late-night poetry reading or catching a train to some political event. I could not stop for the minutiae of motherhood, I told myself when the world itself was like a sick child—hungry, homeless, crazed with material dreams—and in desperate need of advocacy. Mother love? No Pampers or strained peaches for me.[43]

But as a result of so many feminists of the 1970s becoming mothers *despite* the movement's anti-maternal bent, the feminist movement's stance on motherhood began to change. Instead of seeing motherhood itself as the source of women's oppressions, feminists realized that it was the way women in Western cultures were forced to mother—in isolated domestic units, without financial rewards or social status—that often made this wonderful and important experience so harrowing. More recently, Western feminists have also sought to re-vision pregnancy, not as a medical condition, but as a spiritual one with implications for the pregnant woman's selfhood and her relationship with her fetus and child.

Foremost among these has been Dr. Naomi Lowinsky. In her book *The Motherline*, Naomi Lowinsky described all the wonderfully strange and unique aspects of pregnancy:

When a woman becomes a mother her world changes from the inside out. She is shaped from within by the child's development. Boundaries between herself and her baby are blurred as her body and awareness shift to embrace the unknown child. Yet, the one she is bearing, intimate of intimates, sharer of blood and of bodily secretions, is unknown to her . . . her consciousness is being woven by her experience of the pregnancy. She is creating and being created, forming and being formed.[44]

Regis Dunne believes that the significance of pregnancy for women is its involvement "of the woman's whole body, a sharing of her life's substance, in a close bodily relationship, in the most intimate form of human communication, for nine months. For the mother, this may also be an experience of self discovery, but certainly she is the source of the initiation of self in the child."[45]

The views of Lowinsky and Dunne are echoed by the women I interviewed who describe pregnancy as being a unique human relationship between beings who are both interconnected and interdependent. Pro-choice Carmen, for instance, said, "When you are pregnant, you and the baby are a unit. A woman [who is] pregnant is *more* than a woman who is not pregnant. It's not you *and* the baby: the two of you are a single unit."

When I was pregnant I recall this constant—yet almost imperceptible feeling—of splitting into two. It was this process of becoming both someone different, and someone *else*, that left me feeling both vulnerable (who was the person I had been?) and almost preternaturally powerful (I was participating in the creation of and holding under my skin something that would be my child!). I loved the idea that my child had come into being hearing my heartbeat and my voice, yet the agony I felt over my ballooning belly made me aware of how much my self-image and self-esteem were caught up in the view I had of myself when I looked in the mirror. I remember thinking that there was a reason why the pregnancy needed to destroy my previous sense of self, for I could no longer be the same person after the baby was born: because I would then be both a woman who had gestated and given birth to a baby, and a mother who would evermore be responsible for the care of the child I had created. But as necessary as my increasingly slippery sense of self was, it made me feel vulnerable. If I was no longer myself, but not yet a mother, then who was I? The answer—a pregnant woman— was of little comfort because I had no idea, and lacked any cultural examples, of what a pregnant woman did, or was. I thought that perhaps the baby's coming to being in the center of my body was preparing my psyche for the birth, when he or she would displace me at the center of my emotional world. This blurriness between my needs and the baby's needs—between who I was and who the baby was—would be the necessary precondition for the inevitable sacrifices the early years would entail.

In *Of Woman Born*, possibly the first in-depth feminist analysis of women's experience of pregnancy and motherhood, Adrienne Rich wrote:

In pregnancy I did [not] experience the embryo as decisively internal in Freud's terms, but rather, as something inside and of me, yet becoming hourly and daily more separate, on its way to becoming separate from me and of itself . . .

Far from existing in the mode of "inner space," women are powerfully and vulnerably attuned both to "inner" and "outer" because for us the two are continuous, not polar.[46]

### The Pregnant Relationship

The feto-maternal bond [is] established at the physical and metaphysical level. The mechanism of this bonding process is not fully understood in scientific terms, but women know it by experience, and know it to be important, to them and to their children.          —REGIS DUNNE[47]

Far from denying the importance of pregnancy in creating a mean- ingful relationship between herself and her fetus, it is the impor- tance of this relationship to the woman that forms the basis of her decision to continue the pregnancy and become a mother, or to have an abortion. Pregnancy, in other words, is the process through which a woman's "own" child is created and, consequently, the process though which the fetus takes on meaning—as a being that could become the woman's child. However, to say that the fetus is valuable to the woman as a being that could be her child is very different from agreeing with the anti-choice view that the fetus is *intrinsically* and *independently* valuable. The former view is decidedly feminist, valuing women's experience of pregnancy and making it the cornerstone of a women-centered abortion ethic. The latter—which sees the pregnant woman as a fetal container that contributes nothing to pregnancy but a "location" for a tiny, autonomous "baby" to grow into a larger version of itself—is profoundly anti-feminist.

Because it is the fetus's relational qualities that women value—its role as the woman's developing child-to-be—women consider the rectitude of their abortion decisions in terms of their impact on themselves and the fetus as a unit. Just as pregnancy interconnects their present, so will birth intertwine them for the rest of their lives. When women consider the futures of their fetuses, their understanding of the dependency of babies and children ensures that they do not conceive of this future abstractly, but as being intertwined with their own. Ethicist Stephen Ross gave a good explanation of exactly how this works:

Choosing to bring the fetus to term . . . [is] choos[ing] to *have our child*. If, as most parents do, we allow the fetus to live, we may well be doing so with the anticipation of bringing someone into the world with whom we are then quite closely bound. And this possibility (or for most, inevitability) must enter into how we think of the fetus. Hence, intense long range concern over all that awaits the object of our efforts once the physical dependency of pregnancy ends makes sense here . . .[48]

Pro-choice Gillian's words provide a good example of how this sort of understanding of the maternal–fetal connection shaped a past decision to abort: "I was thinking about the baby too. I never considered adoption, but I thought definitely for the baby. I didn't want it. How much more can you think about the baby [than that] it was going to have a miserable life because I didn't want it?"

All the pro-choice women I spoke with, and most of those who were anti-choice, agreed that decisions about pregnancy were women's—and women's alone—to make. The women's views on this question were asserted most strongly when it became clear that ectogenesis had the potential to give men equal control in decisions about the ultimate fate of the fetus. The vast majority of women interviewed, however, maintained that whether or not their fetuses remained in their bodies, the final say on the fate of the fetuses rightfully belonged to them. Pro-choice Margot explained why:

The man is not in the situation where he *has* to make a decision [about the pregnancy], whereas [the woman] does. So it's an unequal situation. Some men do feel a responsibility [for a pregnancy] . . . but the difference is always that he does not become pregnant . . . if a female chooses not to do anything at all, then there are consequences . . . She carries the pregnancy through and becomes a mother. So for her, it's a decision that she can not get away from. For him, it's a decision he actually doesn't have to make. He can just choose to ignore it. A woman can not choose to ignore it.

The other reason the women interviewed thought the abortion decision was rightfully the pregnant woman's to make was their conviction that *no one else* had the necessary moral authority to make these decisions the way they should be made. That it was only the pregnant woman who would make the most careful and caring decisions and that she was the only one who knew all the variables that must be considered. These beliefs, which affirm the moral agency of women, contrast sharply with those espoused by the anti-choice movement. Pro-choice Charity was clear, for example, that the pregnant woman's position on continuing the pregnancy was the only one that mattered because she was the only one who really *cared* about all the lives and issues involved: "My decision to have an abortion would be the decision I made to care for the child within me. My decisions will affect my child in a more humane manner, because I've got my child's interests at heart. And that's why I'd decide to terminate, for that child's sake."

And, as we've already seen, pro-choice Carey also emphasized the caring nature of the abortion decision: "The whole handling of the abortion issue is wrong. I've had an abortion and it was an incredibly painful experience. My decision was not a callous one: it was not unthought about, it was not clear, and it certainly wasn't indifferent."

While women were to be trusted, scientific technology was not. Pro-choice Jacinta insisted that any baby grown artificially—outside the body of its mother—could never be "psychologically normal":

JACINTA: I wouldn't believe that something couldn't happen to that fetus. I would be worried about what would happen to the fetus, during extraction, and once it gets put in the machine, and once it gets to be nine months old. That fetus would, in fact, end up as a baby with a problem.

LC: Why?

JACINTA: Because the technology may go wrong. During the extraction, during the growth of the fetus in the machine. Because eight weeks to nine months is a long time and things have got to go right. I would be concerned that the technology was not perfect, and I would want it to be perfect.

Pro-choice Carey expressed her trust in "natural" pregnancy as against an artificial one: "A pregnancy in the womb results in a child that is whole, that is nourished emotionally, spiritually, and mentally. How do you guarantee that a child will get this if you attach it to some technology?"

Anxiety about a child's well-being, in both the short- and long-term, is clearly behind pro-choice Lisa's joke that an artificially gestated fetus "couldn't even do re-birthing!"

Pro-choice women were suspicious not only of medical technology but of the medical profession that controls it. Pro-choice Lisa minced few words on this topic: "I find it pretty terrifying, doctors having that much power. My work actually involves a lot of technology. I see people at the end of their lives, and I don't like the power doctors have. Giving them that sort of power at the start of life? It's not something I'd ever want them to have."

Pro-choice Carey agreed: "I have a great deal of concern because the male doctors controlling it don't understand anything about the birth process, so they approach birth from a technological point of view. They don't look at things from an emotional and spiritual point of view. For this, you need a woman's perspective."

It was not only pro-choice women who saw themselves as the rightful decision makers in all matters of pregnancy. Most anti-choice women did too, and for the same reasons as their pro-choice counterparts: they were the ones who could be trusted because they really cared:

NELLIE: You can't trust science, anything could go wrong, putting [the fetus] at the mercy of doctors.

NATASHA: But things could go wrong naturally too.

NELLIE: Yes, but at least you haven't given it away, exposed it to even more.

Similarly, distrust of ectogenetic technology and the medical profession was not confined to pro-choice women. Anti-choice Janet clearly thought that she would provide better protection for her fetus than the medical profession: "If you put the fetus into an ectogenetic womb, I would worry that the medical profession wouldn't look after it properly. That they would do something to it and it wouldn't be all right. That it wouldn't be looked after the way it was with me before I handed it over."

Anti-choice Grace also feared that the doctors would "eventually say we can't afford to have all these babies stuck in these ectogenetic wombs, and will just quietly turn off the machines."

The ectogenetic womb was not seen as an answer to the problem of abortion. All the women interviewed agreed that if a child was to be born, pregnancy was a non-negotiable part of a woman's responsibility to that child. An ethical woman wouldn't off-load her gestational responsibilities to an artificial womb, or to anything or anyone else for that matter. For these women, pregnancy grants women sole responsibility for the fetus because the pregnant woman will be the mother of the child the fetus will become. It is the unique relationship between mother and fetus created by pregnancy that forms the cornerstone of women's responsibility-based abortion ethic.

## The Importance of Intentions

There were a number of criteria the women I interviewed had for an ethical abortion. A key one was that the woman didn't *intend* to become pregnant—it was accidental. In the quote below, pro-choice Charity's struggle with the case of a female athlete who purposefully became pregnant to aid her performance demonstrates the inability of feminist claims about "choice" and "control" to capture meaningful ethical distinctions between women's pregnancies, and their abortions:

> I've heard about female athletes getting pregnant because the hormones that are released make them better athletes. I can't remember how far into the pregnancy they have to be, but it made them perform better . . . I thought, "Well, God, they're still in complete control of their bodies" . . . but I still have a bit of a problem with it morally. But I can't figure out why, because the woman is in control . . ."

For all the women I interviewed, a woman's intention in becoming pregnant and her view of pregnancy were key indicators of the morality of her choice to abort. The vast majority of women found the idea of using pregnancy as a means to another end completely repugnant. Firstly, it fails to, in pro-choice Carey's words, "honor" pregnancy as "the phenomenal creation of life." For pro-choice Frances, what gets left out is the "emotional" and "spiritual" aspects of the pregnancy: "You have a relationship. If I was pregnant, I imagine I'd be thinking about my child. Some people name it before it's born, and at one time pregnant women weren't supposed to look at ugly things because it was supposed to harm the fetus."

The other problem with this sort of pregnancy, pro-choice women believed, was the intentions of the female athlete. For pro-choice Janine, getting pregnant with the wrong intentions "trivializes human life. While we're saying we'd like the right to make the decision to have an abortion, we don't think it's a light matter, like sweeping out some fluff or some dirt."

Pro-choice Jacinta, who used to work as an abortion counselor, agreed that the pregnancy and abortion of the athlete posed serious moral problems:

> I see people who repeatedly get pregnant because they don't use contraception. I don't think that they don't use contraception deliberately, it's just something in their make-up or mental attitude that is preventing them from using it at all, or using it properly. There are a lot of different reasons why people don't use contraception properly, reasons not always recognized by the people themselves. But to deliberately get pregnant to win a race? That's off.

Pro-choice Margot agreed: "My initial reaction is yuck. Because it's the deliberate creation of potential life with the deliberate intention of destroying it. It's the deliberateness about it that is off-putting. Mostly when abortion happens, it's the result of non-deliberate action."

One of the interview scenarios asked the women if they would abort an established pregnancy to win a trip to the city hosting the Olympic Games. For pro-choice Annette, her relationship with the fetus would be reason enough to rule out having an abortion for this reason: "I would have made the commitment to that child. And that would be a commitment I made with strength."

Unsurprisingly, anti-choice women agreed with pro-choice women that there is something wrong with a woman using pregnancy as a means to an end, and then seeking an abortion. Anti-choice Lenore, for instance, deplored the deliberateness of the athlete's actions: "It's quite revolting. Deliberately having a child so you can kill it."

Like Annette, anti-choice Karen found intentional conception and abortion morally repugnant because it fails to acknowledge the value of the pregnant woman's relationship with the fetus: "It's saying babies are replaceable . . . I don't think life should be that cheap. 'oh well, got rid of that one, I'll just have another one.'"

For pro-choice women, the feminist contention that the only requirement for an ethical abortion is that a woman freely chooses it was simply not enough. For these women, a particular abortion would only be seen as ethical if the woman became pregnant by accident, and if she considered the state of being pregnant—whether her final choice was for abortion or motherhood—a privileged and sacred one. In addition, pro-choice women felt it necessary that, in her decision-making, the woman consider the fetus not as an autonomous cosmonaut but as a vulnerable and dependent creature who had the capacity to become her child.

While anti-choice women largely disapproved of abortion, they agreed with pro-choice women that the way a woman becomes pregnant, and the way she thinks about pregnancy, are necessary things to know in making a moral assessment of an aborting woman's decision. Women should view pregnancy as an important responsibility, and not intentionally become pregnant unless they intend to mother. They also believed that the moral framework within which women make decisions about pregnancy should include an understanding of pregnancy as a relationship and should value the fetus as the woman's could-be child.

## When Anti-choice Women Favor Choice

Most people have heard of the "hard cases"—those cases of pregnancy in which attempts to deny a woman an abortion become truly obscene: when the pregnant woman's life is at risk, or when she is the victim of rape or incest. Many will remember the international outrage sparked in 1992 by the Irish High Court's refusal to allow a fourteen-year-old rape victim to travel to Europe for an abortion. Of course, if conception is the start of human life, and all humans have "a right to life," no exception can be made for such cases. After all, *how* the fetus is conceived has no bearing on its status as a person. But Janet Hadley tells how disturbed many Irish were when they realized the full impact of the prohibitionist laws governing their country:

In their sympathy for the girl, people realized what a black-and white code on abortion they had voted for. Men and women looked at their daughters, nieces, sisters, who could now be imprisoned in the constitution of Ireland: "If 'X' was my daughter . . . ," they said to each other, and saw that abortion was not that simple.[49]

Certainly, if the hard cases are tests of the consistency of anti-choice views, most of the anti-choice women I interviewed—like much of the Irish public—failed. Anti-choice Maria said that if she was "in danger of dying, I'd put my own life first."

Anti-choice Natasha also softened her anti-choice stance when it came to pregnancy as a result of rape: "If I was raped, I would seriously consider abortion. Because I don't know if I could have the baby with all that anger. I don't know how I'd react to it."

Anti-choice Sarah, on the topic of incest, spoke for a number of the women: "You can't really expect an adolescent incest victim to carry a pregnancy right through, destroying her body as she's doing it. That baby wasn't one born out of love, it was born out of fear and sickness. So there is no love there for that baby."

Anti-choice women used two strategies to deal with the holes the "hard cases" threaten to poke in their positions. Some argued that such cases were statistically insignificant or "trumped up" (presumably by pro-choice forces). Rare or false enough, in other words, not to count as evidence against their anti-choice beliefs. Mary and Susan tried to dismiss the importance Sarah placed on the rape of the young Irish girl:

SARAH: I'm anti-abortion but I'm also, there are situations where you, say for example the girl in Ireland who was raped and everything like that . . .

MARY: Was that true?

SUSAN: That's right, I think that was a big set-up.

MARY: I do too.

As Sarah persisted in arguing in favor of abortion for girls pregnant as a result of incest, Susan continued to insist such cases were too rare to force her to re-think her anti-choice beliefs:

SARAH: At eleven or twelve, even sixteen, they don't understand pregnancy as a baby growing up in them, just as an act of violence that's been taken upon them. There is no love for that baby, they don't love it at all. There is just the pain of bearing . . .

SUSAN: This is a rare case though.

SARAH: To be truthful, an abortion is warranted in that case, but for no other because there have been cases where girls have become pregnant this way, had the baby, and then got pregnant again as a result of incest. You've had to deal with it, to see that it's a very real situation. And it definitely happens, time and again, it's just terrible.

SUSAN: I just wonder what the statistics really are.

SARAH: They're very high.

SUSAN: Because statistics can be made to lie.

The other anti-choice strategy was to hold fast to the claim that abortion was always wrong, but that in rare circumstances a woman who chose one could not be *blamed*. This tactic was the one Susan finally adopted:

Say you were starving, dying of hunger. To steal is morally wrong, isn't it? But to steal when you are very, very hungry for your family? It's morally wrong, but who could blame you for it? There are situations [where the woman would not be to blame], but you just don't talk about it. Sometimes it's up to an individual.

The fact that anti-choice women do not see abortion as an unacceptable moral choice in all circumstances strongly suggests that it is the motives and intentions of aborting women, not the destruction of fetal life, that is at the heart of what these women find so wrong about abortion. If this were not the case, anti-choice women would find women who have abortions blameworthy no matter how they got pregnant, because the status of the fetus is unchanged by the circumstances of its conception.

What this means is that, for the most part, the views of anti-choice women on what makes an abortion ethical *are not very much different* from those of pro-choice women. For both groups, pregnancy must be unintentional and must be valued by the woman as, to use Carey's words, the phenomenal creation of life. The woman must also value the fetus as her particular child-to-be. What was different about pro- and anti-choice women's abortion morality, however, was their different perspective on the trustworthiness of women.

## Can Women Be Trusted?

While agreeing that the aborting woman's motivations and intentions are the key to making a moral assessment of her abortion, pro- and anti-choice women then proceeded to make radically different assumptions about the motives and intentions of the vast majority of women having abortions. For pro-choice women, the assumption was that, most of the time, most women's intentions were good. This assumption was behind Charity's distress at the behavior of the female athlete: "It just doesn't seem to fit in with what a woman is about and what we're capable of. We're still talking about life here, and it goes against life somehow. It's really hard to put it in tangible terms."

If a woman were to make such a decision—like deciding to have an abortion to win a free trip to the Olympics—Jacinta believed this was proof positive she'd make a bad mother: "If a woman did that, I would have a real concern about how she's going to treat her child were it to be born."

But for anti-choice women, the motives and intentions of most women, most of the time, were not to be trusted. Many of them seemed to believe that unplanned pregnancies simply did not happen to women who acted responsibly.

I should have taken responsibility before the baby was created. It's my fault, not the baby's fault. I have no right to kill the baby because I was irresponsible. (Nellie)

Abortion just isn't something I would even contemplate. I just don't believe in it at all. I think there are other ways, not becoming pregnant in the first place, which would mean abortion wouldn't have to be the issue it is. (Mary)

While anti-choice women seem to be castigating women for having unplanned pregnancies, what really concerns them is that women in this situation do not choose to become mothers. Many of them had personally experienced an unplanned pregnancy—pregnancies which they had chosen to bring to term. While discussing one of several unplanned pregnancies, anti-choice Susan noted that "a lot of people in the world wouldn't be here if they were planned and really wanted."

The problem for anti-choice women is not only that women who have abortions don't choose motherhood, but that their decisions to have abortions are made for all the "wrong" reasons. For anti-choice women—and one cannot help but be reminded here of the "heartless" women described by Wolf in what she claims was her "passionately pro-choice" *New Republic* article—the world is full of women who prefer their careers, their skiing trips, or their holidays in Europe to being pregnant and having babies.[50] Anti-choice Charlotte said she knew "of one woman who had an abortion because it was going to interfere with her skiing trip. The pregnancy was just an inconvenience to her."

Anti-choice Marybeth agreed: "Too often women have abortions for reasons of convenience: just for convenience, for money, for having a good time."

Many anti-choice women were also of the opinion that bad

abortion decisions were good indicators of women who would make bad mothers. Susan put it this way:

Let's say I abort this child for convenience. My child will then feel that my attitude toward them is "Oh well, whenever it's not convenient, I forget you because what is most important is for me to do my thing." Children aren't silly. It's not what you say, it's the attitude you have toward them. My children are my life. If I have to make a choice, I choose in favor of my children.

While they disagreed about the morality of abortion, pro-choice and anti-choice women largely agreed on the way abortion should be morally judged. While the fetus figured centrally for all the women, its importance sprang from its current relationship with the pregnant woman and its status as the woman's could-be child. The way women conceived of this relationship, and the actions they took in regard to it, were of central moral importance. It was from this woman-centered perspective that women, not abortions, were being judged.

● ● ●

The parting of the ways for pro- and anti-choice women comes when they assess the trustworthiness of other women. While pro-choice women generally trust that most aborting women are acting morally, anti-choice women are highly suspicious of most women's motivations for seeking abortion. As we shall see in the next chapter, this pattern of agreement and disagreement is not restricted to women's views on pregnancy, but extends to their views of motherhood itself.

# · 5 ·

# The Good Mother

There is only one reason I've ever heard for having an abortion: the desire to be a good mother. Women have abortions because they are aware of the overwhelming responsibility of motherhood.

— DR. ELIZABETH KARLIN,
*director of the Women's Medical
Center in Madison, Wisconsin*[1]

It is startling how similar women's views are of what a good mother is, and what she does. I have found this not only among women I have interviewed for this research, but in later interviews with women on the subject of parenting. I should not have been so astonished. Since the 1950s, when motherhood was redefined from a biological fact (mothers were women who had children) to the task of nurturing and protecting children (a job at which women could succeed or fail), Western cultures like Australia, the United States, and Britain have rigidly defined what a mother should feel, act, and even look like.

In *Of Woman Born*, lesbian feminist poet and author Adrienne Rich describes Western cultures' view of good mothers as "beneficent, sacred, pure, asexual and nourishing," and maternal love as "quite literally selfless." Susan Brownmiller, feminist author of the runaway bestseller on rape *Against Our Will*, has noted in a more recent book about femininity that to be a good *woman*, Western cultures require women to be good *mothers:*

Love of babies, any baby and all babies, not only one's own, is a celebrated and anticipated feminine emotion, and a woman who fails to ooh and ahh at the snapshot of a baby or cuddle a proffered infant in her arms is instantly suspect. Evidence of a maternal nature, of a certain innate competence when handling a baby or at least some indication of maternal longing, becomes a requirement of gender.[2]

In a study of 150 suburban mothers in Sydney, feminist researcher Betsy Wearing found that the extremely diverse group of women she interviewed shared five "principles of motherhood": motherhood is an essential part of womanhood; motherhood is hard but rewarding work; a "good" mother puts her children first; young children need their mothers in constant attendance; mothering is an important but low-status job.

Wearing also found that most women agreed on the following definition of a "good" mother:

A "good" mother is one who is always available to her children; she gives time and attention to them, listens to their problems and questions and guides them where necessary. She cares for them physically . . . and emotionally by showing them love. She is calm and patient, does not scream or yell or . . . smack . . . The cardinal sin of motherhood with its associated guilt is to lose one's temper with a child. Self control should be exercised at all times. Even in extenuating circumstances such as when a baby screams with colic for days or when the mother has no emotional or physical support in her task, she must at all times be in complete control of her own emotions.[3]

The women in a small (unpublished) study I conducted—all expecting their first child in a matter of months—rattled off a similarly challenging list of required attributes for a woman to qualify as a "good" mother:

A good mother is someone who knows the individual needs of her children. She's there for her kids when they need her, treats them as individuals, and knows what each one needs. (Karen)

A good mother makes time to be with her children and when she is with them gives them as much love as she can, and expresses interest in them. She must have respect for herself so that they see her as a role model and have respect for themselves. (Janet)

My mother was a good mother because she was always thinking about other people . . . She was always there when I needed her. When she worked full time she was always up in the morning with all our breakfasts and lunches made . . . Her attention was always on us. (Theresa)

When women fail to meet these high—dare I say, unrealistic—expectations of themselves as mothers, the result can be excoriating guilt. In a 1994 study of ninety Melbourne women, the researchers found that women labeled themselves "bad" mothers if they were unable—at all times—to be "patient, calm, understanding, loving and attentive to their children's needs." Because the authors of the study discovered no evidence that women's expectations of themselves had changed one iota since the mid-1970s, they found well-known writer and feminist Phyllis Chester's questioning of a woman about the nature of good motherhood to still be—however depressingly—highly relevant:

"A good mother is nothing like me," [the woman] said. "A good mother always knows what to do, and does it well, without complaining, without yelling, without manipulating anyone. A good mother uses her power to protect her children from all harm. A good mother has healthy, happy, wonderful children. A good mother is nothing like my mother, or like my grandmother . . ."
    "You're describing a faery goddess and a machine," I interrupt.
    "Yes, maybe I am. But I think that's what a good mother *should* be."[5]

## What Women Want: The Cover Story

A recent survey by *The Age* newspaper of 1000 women living in Melbourne found that 53 percent believed that "a woman should always try to care for her children and not use paid child carers." While women over the age of forty-five were more likely to disapprove of childcare than those aged between eighteen and twenty (63 percent versus 43 percent), women are clearly divided about whether a mother should take on any other job.[6] Here, in many ways, feminists have become stuck. As these recent studies and surveys indicate, feminism has failed to significantly relax both Western culture's and women's own views of what is required of a good mother. This has meant that women's new role of high-achieving career woman has simply been added to the already plentiful demands of "just" being a mother. While many women still attempt to fulfill the role of "supermom," boldly going where no woman has gone before, putting in the long hours and hard work to be a successful career woman and role model for her children *and* being a good mother by providing her children with quality time, endless patience, and nutritious home-cooked meals—many are simply bowing out from exhaustion.

And the demands on working mothers and their partners are growing, as employers pressure men and women to spend more time at the office. According to the Australian Bureau of Statistics, only 35 percent of Australian workers now work a standard 38–40-hour week, and a third of the full-time employees working overtime are doing so for no extra pay. While women are working over 100 hours more per year than they did twenty years ago, men are working an extra 156 hours a year. Don Edgar, a professorial associate at Monash University, says that while many men tell him they'd like to work part-time, when he digs a bit deeper he discovers "they mean forty hours instead of sixty hours a week." And while men do little of the housework or childcare, even if both they and their partners are working full-time, women and children still suffer if the male half of the parental team is regularly getting stuck at the office. Not only do women then have to cope without their partners and with every scrap of housework, they also have to provide all the care for children that are cranky and irritable because they miss their fathers.

The only sane response to all these pressures is to conclude that the family and work demands being made of both women and men are impossible, given the way our world currently works, and to demand such fundamental changes as accessible and free on-site childcare and shorter working hours and higher wages for all (not just the corporate executives). Instead, however, the media and anti-feminists have concluded that the real problem is that too many women are refusing to play wife, and that the blame for that social trend lies at feminism's door. One of the mainstays of efforts to demonize the feminist movement and feminist goals is the regular stories in the media about women who have found happiness after they finally stopped trying to "have it all." Marcia Clark's story—which would sit quite comfortably amidst materials from the Australian Family Association or in a "Women Who Want To Be Women" newsletter, but was actually featured in the Melbourne *Age*—is typical:

Mrs Clarke, 37, was the word processor and personal computer manager for two legal firms and then a contractor for Telecom. She oversaw dozens of operators, millions of dollars of equipment and she worked 80-hour weeks. She was so absorbed in her career that the idea of having a family slowly evaporated. But, as the gloss fell off a life of work, she reconsidered. Before becoming immersed in her career, she had always wanted children . . .

The experience of being full-time mother and homemaker has been unexpectedly rich. "I thought it would be great in a general sense but I didn't realize how fulfilling or enriching it would be." Paid work, a career, by comparison "seems so unimportant." Mothering, on the other hand, "is the most important job in the world."[7]

The media also tends to promote the work of anti-feminists like Catherine Hakim, a research fellow at the London School of Economics. In the middle of 1996, Hakim hit the front pages with her claims that what women *really* want is to look after their homes, their kids, and their men. According to Hakim, assertions that fewer women participate in the workforce than otherwise would if they were actually paid fairly and could get access to proper childcare are myths spread about by a small cadre of "selfish" academic feminists.[8] When many academic feminists questioned Hakim's creative interpretation of the numbers and suggested that social forces might have some influence on the choices women made in relation to work, she went ballistic. She accused them of treating women like "zombies" whose every move is "determined by other actors and social forces." Women, she argued, were making "real" choices in relation to work and were the "authors and agents of their own lives."[9]

The media not only devotes masses of attention to anti-feminist views like Hakim's, it purposefully ignores those facts which support the claims of feminists. For example, Gloria Steinem (citing American statistics that are not too different from those in Australia) has recently condemned the tendency of the media to studiously ignore the fact that women's participation in the workforce continues to grow:

[In 1979 women were 41 percent of the workforce.] By 1990 females of all races made up 57.5 percent of the labor force . . . [with female participation] projected to reach 63 percent by the year 2005. Nonetheless, more media attention has been paid to a statistically insignificant trend of women leaving paid work to raise children—something parents, women or men, should be able to choose, especially in the absence of flexible work schedules and adequate childcare—than to women's positive reasons for staying in the paid labor force.[10]

## Women's Experience of Motherhood: Some Facts

In contrast to the simplicity of the conservative ideologies promoted by anti-feminists and the media, women's actual experience of motherhood is both complex and contradictory. However, one fact that should leave a lot of women breathing easier is that all the claims made about mothers being the only ones able to provide the right sort of care for small children are ripe for challenge. An American study by the National Institute of Child Health and Human Development found no indications that placing children in care with someone other than their mother caused any damage to the relationship between mother and child, regardless of the quality or type of childcare, or the age of the child when they enter care.[11] Of course, as anthropologist Sheila Kitzinger has pointed out, traditional cultures have long known that when the responsibility of childcare is shared, both mothers and children benefit:

When a mother is the sole person to look after a child, who is completely dependent on her, acute sensitivity to her approval may be the result. She represents love, and if this is withdrawn the child has no one else to love it. We tend to think of this as normal, but in most other societies a child does not need the mother's love so unconditionally. There are others who can love and rear the child. Women in peasant societies are often deeply shocked when they learn that in the West a mother may reject, neglect or batter a child. In traditional societies there are always others watching over the care that a woman gives her baby, helping with chores and sharing responsibility.[12]

Drawing conclusions about women's experience of motherhood is difficult not only because one woman's experience differs from another's, but because the same woman's experiences change from hour to hour. A recent study by researchers from the University of Melbourne of 790 new mothers found that 59 percent of women reported not having time to pursue their own interests, 57 percent did not have an active social life, 55 percent needed a break from the demands of the child.[13] Despite the attempts of the media to use Marcia Clark stories to convince women that the difficult jobs they do as mothers are valued by society, women are not fooled. Refusing to pay women or accord them status for mothering (mothering is not considered a real job) and isolating them in single family houses without the company of other adults ensures that many women who mother suffer a loss of self-esteem. The University of Melbourne study found that 55 percent of women had less confidence since they'd become mothers. One woman explained it this way: "I find after I've had the children that I sort of lack a lot of self-esteem too. You feel like, really there's nothing else in the world except you and the baby and it just—it's all there is. All of a sudden you think, oh, there's gotta be more to—there was more to life than me and a baby, and now there's not."[14]

A study of forty married women living in London and mothering at least one child found that while some women did enjoy the work of childcare, a high proportion did not. These women experienced "the endless stream of daily tasks—bathing, dressing, feeding, putting their children to bed at night, tidying up after them, responding to their demands for attention—as an exhausting and predominantly frustrating and irritating experience."[15]

Yet despite the pressures and frustrations, women also find motherhood incredibly fulfilling. The Melbourne *Age* survey, for instance, found that 44 percent of women interviewed nominated mother as their most important role, with those naming wife, partner, or girlfriend as their most important role coming in a poor second at 28 percent. Similar results were found in a 1991 survey of British women conducted by the progressive paper the *Guardian*.[16] After the birth of her first child when she was thirty, journalist Catherine Ford wrote:

I had borne a child, and I was now a mother. I had become someone I didn't recognize. I cried more easily and more often than my baby did. I was open to everything around me in a way I wasn't used to. I had somehow come undone, a bit like the once neat vagina I had that was now only holding its shape with the help of stitches. I was a person who felt. I was not in control of myself.
This, I knew, was the start of my real life.[17]

Single mother Dorothy McNeill, who worked part-time, also said mothering had been her most important role: "Parenting was my most fulfilling role, and I'm quite proud of how my sons turned out."[18]

## What Women Really Want

So it seems that in women's lives work and motherhood, like most things in life, are sources of both extreme stress and extreme satisfaction: a mixed bag, so to speak. When Catherine Hakim claimed that what women *really* want is to stay at home, many feminists argued that it was impossible to know what women *really* want, given the impact of our culture's ideology of motherhood on their needs and desires. What "really" is supposed to mean in these sorts of arguments is "naturally," and what Hakim is claiming is that women's desires not to work are a result of their "natures" (or the biological make-up that God gave them). Of course, what *really* makes such claims stupid is the impossibility, in the real world, of separating out human needs derived from human biology and those born of cultural conditioning. As feminist scientists Ruth Lowe and Marian Hubbard put it: "people's biological and social experiences are intimately interwoven and build upon each other in such multiple ways that it is impossible to sort them out."[19]

It has been part of the agenda of the "new right" (really the old right in new suits) to demonstrate that a woman's "nature"—a nature defined as nurturing, passive, and maternal—is based in female biology. According to Hubbard and Lowe, the choice of this strategy by social conservatives is no coincidence:

For someone who opposes social change, it is convenient to believe that social inequality is rooted in biology. In that case, one can argue that major changes in the social and economic order would require not major political changes—which, in principle, can be brought about rather quickly—but profound changes in human biology, which are difficult to achieve and may take eons.[20]

The feminists who argued against Hakim made standard feminist claims about the impossibility of knowing what women *really* want from what they *say* they want. According to these feminists, this is because women are swamped by our culture's ideologies about what real—read feminine—women *should* desire. Academics call this point of view, which essentially argues that women are not born but made, the "cultural constructivist" perspective. It is summarized here by feminist anthropologists Sherry Ortner and Harriet White-head: "What gender is, what men and women are, what sort of relations do or should obtain between them—all of these notions do not simply reflect or elaborate upon biological givens, but are largely products of social and cultural processes."[21]

It is in the area of motherhood that arguments about the radical influence of culture on women's needs and desires have been taken to their logical extremes. Feminists like Robyn Rowland and Gena Corea have made their names insisting that whatever women say, most don't *really* (there is that word again) want to be mothers. Essentially, Rowland believes that it is impossible to know if a woman's desire for motherhood is "real," because in the patriarchal pro-natalist culture in which we live, women's desire for maternity is mandated:

Ideologies, or belief systems, support . . . [patriarchal] social structures so that the less powerful come to believe that the relative differences in power are natural and acceptable. Men as a social group work to convince women that they are "naturally" worth less, are "naturally" mothers, and so must "naturally" be responsible for domestic labour. People develop within these ideologies to which they are so accustomed that they do not question them. Some of the "control" myths about women are: that they should be selfless and self sacrificing . . . and are in a position of lesser power because of a "natural" inclination. Moreover, to be a good woman," [they] . . . really ought to be a mother.[22]

My point is that if it is tripe to say that what women really want is *solely* based in their biological natures, it is also tripe to argue that *nothing* women say they want can be trusted because their needs have been entirely conditioned by the patriarchy. While feminists must continue to work for a world that is as free as possible from economic and social pressures on women to conform to particular models of womanhood, it is both insulting and unworkable to dismiss the desires of women living in the real world as simply the result of cultural brainwashing. Despite the powerful influences of culture, feminists must consider women's choices about motherhood —and anything else in fact—to be worthy of respect. The fact is that *all* decisions, including reproductive ones, are a complex mixture of biological and cultural influences. And no matter how their needs are formed, women experience them as powerfully real. Feminist authors Lynda Birke, Susan Himmelweit, and Gail Vines put it this way:

> Understanding where a need comes from does not remove it . . . [A]ll needs and desires are socially produced, whether or not, like feelings about reproduction, they centre on a process that has some biological content too . . . [T]here may be strong pressure, from ideology or even from instincts, on women to be mothers in our society, but we are all subject to pressure in many areas of our lives and that does not make us incapable of making choices or the decisions that we take any less worthy of respect.[23]

The bottom line is that women must be seen to be making real choices for them to be considered moral agents. It is only when people have choices about what they say and do that they can be praised or blamed. This is a familiar concept in the judicial system where only those who are "competent" are held accountable for their behavior. Ironically, feminists support anti-feminist claims about women's diminished moral capacities when they propose or support arguments that dismiss women's desires as nothing but the result of patriarchal brainwashing.

## The Good Mother and Adoption

Almost all the women I interviewed, no matter what their views were on abortion, held that "good" mothers have a variety of responsibilities to their fetuses and their children—responsibilities that spring from the pregnant relationship. These women believed it was up to them to gestate "their own" fetuses and to raise "their own" children to adulthood. If a child was to come into this world, in other words, it was its mother's responsibility to gestate that child in her own body and to raise it after birth. A "good" woman would not off-load the responsibility of pregnancy to an artificial womb nor the responsibilities of motherhood to another woman. While a woman may be entitled to the title of mother if she is only the genetic mother of the child, or if she carries the child for the full term of a pregnancy, she is only a *good* mother if she accepts and rejoices in the role of nurturer and parent of her fetuses and children.

These beliefs obviously raise some questions about the practice of adoption. The accepted view of adoption is that because it saves the life of the fetus, moral women should choose it over abortion. In addition, women who give away their children to "people who can't have their own"—as in the case of both adoption and surrogacy—get lots of kudos in our culture for their "sacrifice." According to many relinquishing mothers and their lost children, however, the practice of adoption has given them nothing but pain and sorrow: "The feeling of loss has been strong for eighteen years—it was as though she died, only worse, she was out there somewhere. I don't even have the right to wonder or ask how she is . . . [but] I do wonder, cry, and ask."[24]

An Australian Institute of Family Studies report on 213 mothers who relinquished a child for adoption found that:

The effects of relinquishment on the mother are negative and long-lasting. Approximately half the women reported an increasing sense of loss over periods of up to thirty years. Relinquishing mothers compared to a carefully matched comparison group of women had significantly more problems of psychological adjustment. Relinquishing mothers believed that their sense of loss and problems of adjustment would be significantly eased by knowledge about what had happened to the child they gave away.[25]

Adoption experts Silber and Speedlin call adoption a "psychological amputation" because birth parents "care deeply for the life they create. The decision to relinquish that life for someone else to parent is an unforgettable decision. This decision can result in a lifetime of grief and despair."[26]

One birth mother described that "amputation" as being a far worse experience than illegal abortion:

The physical pain and danger associated with [three illegal] abortions were nothing compared with the agony and lifelong regret I have experienced as a result of adopting out my baby. I have never been able to stop wondering if she's alright. I have never regretted my abortions, but I will regret adopting out my baby for eternity.[27]

In response to claims that the secretive and coercive nature of past adoption practices was the source of many relinquishing mothers' heartache, one anti-adoption activist noted:

Whether we [choose to give up our babies] with free will, whether we choose because we are under pressure, whether we choose because we've agreed to for a whole range of other reasons; no matter how we "choose" to give a child away, it inevitably leaves with us an experience of such vast pain and loss that we are never the same people again.[28]

The majority of studies of relinquishing mothers find that years later "child surrender remains an issue of conflict and intrapersonal difficulty" for these women.[29] Women who have surrendered their children for adoption report problems with their health, their marriages, and their fertility. Looking back on their decision, women who kept their children were more satisfied with their choice than those who relinquished them.[30] Even birth mothers who didn't regret their decision to adopt wanted, in the vast majority of cases, to have some ongoing contact with the child they'd surrendered.

A look at adoption rates shows that birth mothers are voting with their feet—and keeping their children. In the 1970s, 80 percent of babies born to unwed American mothers were placed for adoption. In 1983, that number had plummeted to only 4 percent. In Australia, adoption figures are now at their lowest level, down from 10,000 in the early 1970s to 764 in 1993–94, with most of those children born overseas. In one Australian state, the number of parents applying to adopt is ten times the number of available children. Experts attribute this radical fall in adoption rates to the decreased stigma of abortion and its greater availability as well as a less moralistic view of premarital sexual activity, a high divorce rate (which has made single parenthood commonplace), and a growing acceptance in the community of the feminist movement's demands for women's rights.

In addition to these factors, the introduction in Australia of a pension for single mothers, and an official view that children should remain with their natural family no matter what, have also increased the numbers of women choosing to keep their babies.

Adoption is not only traumatic for the birth mother, adopted children often suffer too. Many experience a feeling of "genealogical bewilderment," the sense of not belonging to the adopted family and of rejection by the natural family. One adoptee, Ferg, described himself in his diaries as an "adoptaholic": "So many of my thoughts, so much of my time, so much of my energy had been directed into the fact that I had been adopted and that I knew no roots. It had just not been a small aspect of my life but a gnawing obsession."[31]

Most adopted children seem to mourn the birth bond rather than the genetic bond, leading them to search firstly, and in many cases only, for their mothers. Like many adoptees, Ferg's primary interest was in finding his mother, not his father. When he saw the birth of his daughter, and the "incredible bond" between her and his wife, he'd wondered "how in hell can a mother let go of her child? And what hell did [my birth mother] go through?"[32]

Suzanne Chick, who wrote a book about her search for her birth mother—well-known author Charmian Clift—was also disinterested in finding her father. For her, the search for her mother was "mystical": "I sensed myself tapping into some universal mother-to-daughter continuum. It stretched back into time: me, my mother Charmian, her mother. And it stretched into the future: my three daughters . . . and their unborn daughters, and theirs after them. Womb to womb to womb."

## Pro-choice Women and Adoption

All the pro-choice women I interviewed ruled out adoption as an option for them. Their primary reason? That giving up a child they had carried for nine months—their "own" child—would simply be too painful:

Having had children, I think it would be very difficult to give a child up for adoption if you'd gone through the pregnancy. (Jacinta)

I'd rather terminate than go through the pregnancy and have to go through the trauma of giving up a child at the end, after giving birth to it. (Charity)

To go through six, seven, eight months of justifying why you're going to give it away when the whole time you're bonding to it yourself? It would make you crazy. I don't know how people could do it, I could certainly never see myself doing it. (Gillian)

Janet Hadley pointed out that women also reject adoption because of concern about the impact of relinquishment on the children they've already got: having "to weigh the emotional impact on those children of seeing their mother carry a pregnancy to term and then 'give the baby away.'"[33]

The pro-choice women interviewed were also crystal clear that people would think they were unmotherly and immoral—and would disapprove of them—for choosing adoption:

People would say, "How on earth could you give up a baby? How could you be so cold and calculating to give up a baby?" (Jacinta)

You've still got to go to work, go shopping, see your friends. They'll all assume you're having a baby because you want to, not because you've made this moral decision that it's wrong to kill the baby. So it's not only what you think, it's the pressures of people around you. (Gillian)

In addition to the emotional pain and social stigma, pro-choice women worried about the pain a child would suffer in not being raised by the person who gestated them—their mother. By severing the relationship established by nine months of pregnancy, and in casting the child into the world without the sense of self bestowed on children raised by their own mothers, these women feared their children would be unable to establish a solid sense of themselves or find happiness. Charity's view on this matter was typical: "I would be frightened of what would happen to them, and that I'd damaged them by not having any influence on them."

The point is that the pregnant relationship is not merely a physical one, but one that provides a social context for the fetus and the child when it is born. Robyn Rowland writes: "One of the things which women understand is that mothering is a relationship, not just between the woman and the child, but between the woman, the child, and a nexus of other people involved in that relationship."[34]

Academic feminist Heather Deitrich agrees:

Particular physical, emotional and social relationships are built within pregnancy . . . Pregnancy and birth are social events as well as biological events. The birth mother gives the child a place, and continuity with a family line. Relinquishment of the child to another family is a social, as well as physical and psychological dislocation and relocation.[35]

## Anti-choice Women and Adoption

> During a pro-life vigil outside Parliament House, I was attacked by
> hard-faced, pro-abortion feminists. One of these angry feminists
> even tried to scratch my face and screamed at me "There is nothing
> in an abortion, I've had seven." No wonder she had lost her
> femininity.          *Anti-choice activist* FRED NILES[36]

When the anti-choice women in my study discussed the problem of
an unwanted pregnancy in abstract terms, the solution they nominated was adoption. Their reasons for preferring adoption to abortion ranged from the dictates of their religion, to the unequivocal
value of "life," to the needs of the infertile:

I'm a practicing Catholic and my religion says abortion is committing a
mortal sin. (Gina)

I would choose adoption because it would give that life a chance somewhere else. (Jamie)

If I couldn't keep the child, I'd give that child up for adoption. The reason
being that I know people who have been unable to have children and
they've always wanted to adopt and I know the joy that gives parents who
aren't able to have a child. (Maria)

But when push came to shove, none of the anti-choice women
really thought a "good" mother would ever give her own child
away. Essentially, anti-choice women thought that while adoption
was the right way for women to deal with unwanted pregnancies in
theory—a position consistent with the anti-choice movement's promotion of adoption as the alternative to abortion—it had little appeal in practice. If any of these women were *themselves* pregnant, in
other words, they would not choose adoption, but instead would
find some way to keep their child. The reasons why relinquishment
was not a real option for these women were almost the exact same
ones given by their pro-choice counterparts: the pain involved for
the woman, and the relationship created between mother and child
by the pregnancy:

MARTINA: I've had two children, and before I had them I would have said I'd choose adoption if faced with an unplanned pregnancy, because I don't believe in abortion. But I couldn't adopt a child either, because you do grow to love it so much. I've had to make that choice, with my second child, because we really couldn't afford it. But I decided to keep my second child because I just couldn't part with it.

LC: So for you—faced with an unwanted pregnancy—the choices in theory are adoption or keeping it, but in reality the only choice is keeping it?

MARTINA: Yes. It was something we talked about, but I just couldn't think of doing it. No, I just think there's too much bonding, it's too hard to do.

MARY: I'd choose adoption as opposed to abortion, but I don't think it would ever come to that. I think I'd probably find a way to bring it up myself.

LC: Why don't you think you'd be able to adopt?

MARY: I don't think I could go through the nine months of being pregnant and have the baby and then give it away.

SARAH: I wouldn't have an abortion. I'd carry that baby, but I wouldn't be able to adopt. I'd find some way to keep that baby.

LC: It's not even imaginable?

SARAH: No. I just wouldn't do it. I know myself, I couldn't give that baby up. I really couldn't.

It is possible that the anti-choice movement counsels women with unwanted pregnancies to choose adoption instead of abortion *precisely because* they know so many women will, in the end, be unable to give up their child after birth, and so will end up "choosing" motherhood. Grace, a pregnancy counselor for the anti-choice movement, said that she advises pregnant women to take a "wait and see" attitude:

There's no doubt that the hormonal changes in your body do things to you. Now, I had sixteen horrible weeks of morning sickness and I thought, I hate this child, I despise this child. But it passes, and once you feel the joy of the first movement, the changes come within your system and your heart. And these changes just continue, and by the time the pregnancy's finished, you might feel differently.

Like their pro-choice counterparts, anti-choice women also feared that—despite adoption's public status as an ethical choice—people would think badly of them if they gave their child away. Says Amanda:

People would see you and there would just be an automatic assumption that you would be keeping the child and the difficulty would be [in] saying, "No, I'm not keeping the child." That's when you'd get the pressure from people. I really don't know if they would accept that you were going to give it up . . . They would think badly of you.

## Mothering Against the Odds: A New Test of Good Womanhood

The availability of abortion has changed the way women look at pregnancy. Instead of something that just comes, so to speak, with the territory, pregnancy is now seen as a positive decision not to abort. While pro-choice women choose abortion as the solution to all the problems of adoption, anti-choice women's opposition to abortion means that their concerns about adoption must be addressed differently. Their solution has been to refashion unwanted pregnancy into a test of a woman's moral character. A woman is good, they say, if she chooses motherhood, and is extra virtuous if she chooses motherhood *despite* or *against* the odds. Says anthropologist Faye Ginsburg:

[In the post-legalization era] the decision to keep the pregnancy despite adverse circumstances becomes an achievement, rather than the inexorable if begrudging fulfillment of a predetermined . . . role. The woman who decides to carry an unwanted pregnancy comes to signify an asserting of a particular construction of female identify . . . in which nurturance, achieved through accepting pregnancy and birth, is of paramount value . . . In the pro-life view, women who choose, in the face of problematic circumstances, to keep an unwanted pregnancy when abortion is a choice, are "truly" female . . . By contrast, women who abort or advocate abortion are marked as "unfemale."[37]

Anti-choice Susan spoke of how difficult it was for her to go on with the pregnancy of her third child so shortly after the birth of her twins:

a year and a half later I had Kristin and then another one after that. Certainly being pregnant so soon again after the twins wasn't easy. My doctor said, "This is a bit soon, would you consider an abortion? You're young, you can have more children." And we were in a difficult situation—my husband was out of work and I was looking after my elderly mother-in-law. But look at her now, she's gorgeous.

Like Susan's experience, Sarah's story emphasizes the moral values of those who raise children in the face of obvious and undeniable hardship:

I knew a couple having their fifth child who had decided to give up the baby for adoption, but once it was born, they just could not give up this child. They were in tears, and it was a very emotional time. They were very certain they were going to give it up, they got the papers and everything. But when I saw them the next day, they just couldn't do it. I was just about in tears myself because I thought there was just so much love between them and they were going to give up their baby. OK, they may have to struggle, but there was just too much love to give up that baby.

## When the "Solution" Is the Problem: Pro-choice Women Reject Ectogenesis

It is the desire of pro-choice women to live according to their ethical codes about what a good mother is and does that leads them to insist upon the deaths of the fetuses they will be unable to gestate and mother themselves. A woman makes an ethical stand when she rejects fetal evacuation (which keeps the fetus alive) or insists upon abortion (which kills the fetus). The desire to bring about the death of one's own fetus, says ethicist Stephen Ross, "is bound up with the most central values [a] person holds: one wants very much to be a certain kind of person, that is, the sort who has children only when able to raise them oneself in an environment one finds right."[38]

Almost all the pro-choice women I interviewed thought ectogenesis was an even less moral choice than adoption, because instead of giving away one's fetus and child to another woman, a pregnant woman was relinquishing her fetus to a machine.

I think it would be wrong for the child to know that it was conceived in a woman's body and then given up to a machine because the woman didn't want it, and then adopted to a couple to raise . . . Unless it is dealt with in a very sensitive way, the child could feel very unwanted. (Jacinta)

If you have a baby at nine months and adopt it to a family, you've got the worry of whether the mother is doing the right thing by "your" baby. But if you put your baby into an ectogenetic womb, you would really worry about how it was being looked after. (Janet)

For many of the women, ectogenesis was rejected simply on the grounds that it was "early adoption." Frances said, "I still wouldn't be able to separate myself from the child I had conceived. It would still be out there somewhere. It's really just adoption before you give birth to the child."

According to Callie, neither adoption nor ectogenesis solved the pregnant woman's problems because, in perpetuating the child's life, its mother's responsibility is also perpetuated: "No matter what you thought, there's life there, and you are responsible. You've put another person on the planet and you will always be responsible for them."

If a good mother raises her own children, then the only way to avoid this responsibility is not to have children in the first place. Time-warping would be the ideal solution for most women considering abortion, since what most of them want is to simply turn the clock back to the time before they were pregnant and there was anyone for whom they were—and would continue to be—responsible. Because this is not possible, pro-choice women believe the most ethical thing they can do is not to bring a child they cannot raise into being in the first place, so they have an abortion.

The critical point is that pro-choice women see abortion as a *preventative* measure. By preventing their child coming into existence in the first place, women believe they have ethically rid themselves of the responsibilities of motherhood. Canadian Holocaust survivor and abortion-service provider Henry Morgentaler believes that women view abortion not as murder but as prevention: "A woman who wants an abortion doesn't want to kill a baby. She doesn't want the product of conception to *become* a baby."[39]

Because neither adoption nor ectogenesis prevents their child from coming into existence, pro-choice women saw these as completely immoral solutions to unwanted pregnancy. The pregnant woman was not gestating and raising her child and so was guilty of abandoning her maternal responsibilities:

My decision to have an abortion would be the decision I made to care for the child that was within me. To put the child in an ectogenetic womb would be more cruel to me than just ending it because it's giving the child no help. It's saying, "Well, it's not my problem." When you have an abortion, you are making a decision about your own body and about that human's life. (Charity)

What all this adds up to is a clear affirmation by pro-choice women that the decision to abort is not primarily a decision to end a pregnancy, but a decision not to become a mother:

When I thought I was pregnant, the choice I had was either to accept involvement in the creation of a valuable human being and the responsibility for growing, rearing, and parenting that human being, or to reject that responsibility. I wouldn't choose adoption or ectogenesis because either I commit to having a child and am therefore responsible for that child's gestational growth and continuing welfare, or decide against parenting and have an abortion. (Annette)

## When the Solution Doesn't Totally Solve the Problem: Anti-choice Women and Ectogenesis

Those who are familiar with the standard arguments for and against abortion are likely to find anti-choice women's rejection of ectogenesis surprising. After all, ectogenesis preserves the right to life of the fetus, doesn't it? Yet the anti-choice women I interviewed were just as unimpressed with ectogenesis as those on the pro-choice side, and for similar reasons. Like pro-choice women, anti-choice women worried that their fetus wouldn't develop normally outside their bodies, that "science" could not be trusted with their fetuses, and that children born from a machine would lack a stable sense of self:

I've been pregnant and I know what it's like to have a baby growing inside of you, it's just the most amazing thing. I would be worried that something would happen to the baby [in the ectogenetic womb] that I could have prevented when it was in its natural environment. (Martina)

You know when they put the baby on the mother's stomach after it's born and there's that bonding moment? I think that probably starts during the pregnancy because the baby remembers its mother's voice and her heartbeat. I don't know how a sterile environment like a capsule would take the place of that. (Charlotte)

With this modern technology, a lot of children might be born who don't have roots and don't know where they come from. There is not the security of the family, and we might end up with children who really don't know what their purpose in life is. (Susan)

The biggest objection anti-choice women had to ectogenesis, however, was that it simply did not solve the real concerns they have about abortion. The artificial womb might save a fetus's life, but anti-choice women agreed with pro-choice ones that this did not make it right for a pregnant woman to put her fetus in one. This demonstrates—as did the position of most of the anti-choice women on abortion in the "hard" cases—that the death of the fetus is not the only problem anti-choice women have with abortion. Rather, these women oppose abortion because abortion happens when a woman says "no" to motherhood. In fact, most of the anti-choice women were incensed by the possibility that a woman who chose ectogenesis might feel she hadn't done anything wrong because she hadn't had an abortion:

> [T]here are always people ready for a cop-out and [putting your fetus in an artificial womb] is an easy cop-out. It negates your responsibility. Even if the fetus can grow in the womb and someone else adopts it and rears it, for that woman it is still a cop-out. A way that she can say, "I haven't had an abortion so therefore I haven't done anything wrong." There [is] something wrong with taking it out of you and sticking it in a machine. (Grace)

> [Women choosing ectogenesis] might see it as a better solution because they wouldn't have as much guilt as if they had an abortion . . . because they haven't actually killed the baby. But [it's still wrong] because they aren't physically doing any more for it . . . Why are all these options, cop-outs I call them, being created anyway? If you can't accept the responsibility of your child, well then . . . (Miranda)

What all this shows is that, like pro-choice women, anti-choice women know that the abortion decision is not essentially about ending a pregnancy but about choosing motherhood. The goal of anti-choice women in supporting a movement that seeks to make abortion illegal is not the preservation of "innocent" fetal life but the conscription of all women who have conceived to motherhood.

## The Motherhood Debate

Perhaps the bitter and divisive "abortion debate" should be renamed the "motherhood debate." Certainly the sharply different views held by pro- and anti-choice women about what priority women should give to motherhood in their lives is at the heart of the conflict over abortion. Their different views lead these women to choose different labels—moral or immoral—for the majority of women who chose abortion. As we have already seen, anti-choice women have a distinct distrust of the motives and intentions of women who seek abortions. This distrust is summarized by the tag they attach to almost all the reasons women have for choosing abortion—"convenience." Women who abort to—in Marybeth's words—avoid the "hassle and inconvenience" of babies are women with the sorts of inadequate value systems that lead them to value the material aspects of life above their roles as mothers. Anti-choice women see motherhood as the only ethical choice for any pregnant woman—regardless of the "expected" or "unexpected" nature of the pregnancy. In their view, a woman who considers a pregnancy or a child "unwanted" simply lacks the right sorts of ideas about motherhood and womanhood. Anti-choice women believe that a good woman is one who primarily values herself as a good mother.

As a consequence, anti-choice women see abortion as a personal affront to their values and life choices. They view it as a decision that derides and belittles both motherhood and those women, like themselves, who have placed it at the center of their lives. They see pro-choice women as being allied with the breed of 1970s feminists who, in their zeal to ensure women's rights to equal pay and opportunities outside the home, tended to ignore or belittle women who were "only" housewives and mothers. The hysteria that followed Hilary Clinton's cookie baking remarks during the 1992 American presidential campaign is dramatic evidence of the continued sensitivity of full-time home-makers to any suggestion that their life choices are undervalued by "career" women. But, according to Australian feminist Eva Cox, feminist disdain for full-time home-makers, if it ever existed, is certainly no more: "Almost everyone who is a mother thinks being a mother is most important. So the idea that women who go to work denigrate the role of mother does not hold up—mothers, regardless of work status, regard mothering as their most important role. This is not the popular mythology."[40]

The power of the mythology means that "feminist" continues to be a favorite anti-choice "insult" directed toward women who choose abortion—shorthand for the most potent slurs that can be hurled at a Western woman: that she is selfish and unfeminine. Rebecca Albury notes:

Pro-life women . . . see terminations as a direct and serious blow against motherhood, the family, Christian values and the lives they've chosen to lead. Right to life women tend to have come from homemaker backgrounds, usually religious . . . and see terminations as something that devalue motherhood and everything they represent.[41]

## Women Who Choose Abortion: The Real Story

Claims that the majority of abortions are had casually by professional women worried about the impact of a baby on their career are false. Most women terminate because they can't afford a child, or don't want to raise one without a father. *New York Times* columnist Mary Kay Blakely, in recalling a conversation she had over lunch with a priest, shows how the "convenience" label makes unwanted pregnancies the responsibility of individual women, rather than society as a whole:

The statistics suggest to him that . . . women chose abortion for their own "convenience." It's convenient for him not to believe that behind the gross number there is that much poverty, that much despair, that much rape, that much incest, that much woman battering. It's easier to believe that the number of abortions each year attests to the immorality of women, thus shifting the responsibility from the culture collectively to women alone.[42]

But taunting aborting women as "selfish" is popular with antichoicers precisely because such taunts tend to hit home. Abortion counselor Antonia Clissa says that women who consider abortion "are very concerned about being considered selfish . . . A lot of this fear of 'being selfish' is very closely tied to women's self-worth, self-esteem and their social conditioning."[43]

The conclusion of feminist Linda Francke's editorial about her article vividly demonstrates the on-going difficulty many women have when they make hard choices based on their own value system:

And it certainly does make more sense not to be having a baby right now— we say that to each other all the time. But I have this ghost now. A very little ghost that only appears when I'm seeing something beautiful, like the full moon on the ocean last weekend. And the baby waves at me. And I wave at the baby. "Of course, we have room," I cry to the ghost. "Of course we do."[44]

Because a woman thinks she did the right thing in having an abortion, doesn't mean she doesn't grieve. According to Antonia Clissa, women forced to make a decision about an unplanned pregnancy grieve no matter what they choose:

If they choose motherhood, there is the grief and loss of the single life, of personal freedom, the end of innocence and beginning of assuming responsibility for their lives and for that of another being. This may come with either a commitment to the relationship or with the ending of the relationship. If they chose to terminate the pregnancy, there is the loss of parenting the potential life . . . Some women may not have any associated grief at the time and may experience it many years later or not at all, but the women I see all seem to share some element of grief . . . whatever decision they make.[45]

What pro-choice women assume, however, is that they, and other women, are entitled to chart their own destiny. While almost all of these women were already mothers or planned to become mothers in the future, they clearly did not see motherhood as a compulsory part of the definition of an ethical woman. Says Frances, for instance:

I'm not sure [childbearing] is a woman's only role. I probably won't engage in that role at all, but that doesn't mean that I don't have an alternative role . . . Having an abortion is not really selfish because I might be considering my parents, the contribution I might make to society if I don't give myself up to childbearing for the next few years. The contribution I can make if I'm not like my younger sister, who had two young children on her own and is draining my parents financially and emotionally and who has only very recently been able to get out and earn her own living. So it's not selfish, you have a wider responsibility to other people—people you know and people you don't know.

While pro-choice women are comfortable with the idea that a women may choose to abort in order to fulfill her individual aspirations, they believe that the needs of everyone who will bear some responsibility for the child should be considered. So, for instance, the life goals of Linda Francke's husband, as well as her own, factored in her abortion decision:

My husband talked about his plans for a career change in the next year, to stem the staleness that fourteen years with the same investment-banking firm had brought him. A new baby would preclude that option.

The timing wasn't right for me either. Having juggled pregnancies and child care with freelance jobs I could fit in between feedings, I had just taken on a full-time job. A new baby would put me right back in the nursery just when our youngest child was finally school age. It was time for *us* . . .[46]

It is critical to note that Linda Francke's choice was consistent with her valuing of herself as a journalist. She would have had to have been a different person, with a different set of values, to have chosen to adopt or keep the child, in the same set of circumstance. Pro- and anti-choice women may well disagree about what values are the "right" ones, but the anti-choice movement's depiction of aborting women as acting without reference to any recognizable ethical values is misleading and untrue. Moral values—some that are similar and some that are different from those of anti-choice women—are undoubtedly governing the decisions pro-choice women make about unwanted pregnancies.

## A Question of Timing

A central aspect of the abortion dispute is timing. While pro-choice women believe there is *still time* for a pregnant woman to ethically refuse to take on the responsibilities of motherhood, anti-choice women believe that, once pregnant, the woman has no choice but to become a mother. Anti-choice women seem to accept a woman's desire to delay or space her pregnancies using birth control, but red flags seem to go up when they contemplate her delaying childbearing *too long* or *forever,* especially for the sake of her career. Once motherhood is no longer a woman's primary objective, she becomes unfeminine in the eyes of anti-choice women and, therefore, immoral.

Of course, imbedded in beliefs about timing are assumptions about the value of human life. So when a pro-choice woman says she thinks early abortion is killing something that is *not yet* her child, implicit in this view is a belief that embryos and fetuses *do not* equal babies. Their reasons for thinking the embryo and the fetus are not the same as a baby are not based on scientific evidence about "when life begins," but on an understanding of the fetus's and child's life—both physically and emotionally, both now and in the future—as inextricably intertwined with their own. Pro-choice Jane put it well:

I think that this society is really screwed up and it hurts people, and [the child to be aborted] would be one less person that gets hurt. I never think of abortion in terms of whether the fetus is a person or not. I know that if I continue the pregnancy and don't miscarry then it will become a person, so whether it's a person when I have an abortion is not an issue for me. The issue is what's going to happen to this kid after it's born.

Alongside their belief that the fetus is not the same as a baby is pro-choice women's view that life has a relative, rather than an absolute, value. Like proponents of euthanasia, these women believe that life is not always better than death. If she will be unable to look after her fetus in utero, and after birth if she will be unable to be a good mother to her could-be child—the pro-choice woman believes her fetus would be better off dead. Far from being a punishment of her could-be child, pro-choice women see abortion as a safeguard against the creation of a child whom she believes would be better off not being born.

What pro-choice women *are not* saying is that if they are, however, unable to provide their child with the life they believe it should have *after* it is born, then it would be all right to kill it. When infanticide came up in several pro-choice interviews, it was roundly condemned by most of the women. It seems that while pro-choice women believe that a woman has a bit of time after she conceives to accept or reject the responsibilities of motherhood, she doesn't have forever. Once she has made a commitment to continue to nurture and bear the fetus and raise the child, to then renege on this commitment without good reason would be wrong. Annette said: "If I'd decided to [have the child], I would have made a commitment to that child, and that's a commitment I made with strength. [Nothing] is going to change that. Once I'd decided to have the child, that's it."

This sort of thinking may also explain why so many women—including an ever-increasing number of pro-choice feminists—are morally uncomfortable with late-term abortions. It is not that the late-term fetus is more "baby-like" than the earlier one, but that it is disturbing to think that the pregnant woman waited so long before deciding *against* the responsibilities of motherhood. When good reasons for why the abortion was delayed are provided (the woman just found out the baby will be seriously handicapped; she had trouble arranging childcare and raising the money to travel interstate or from the country to a regional center for the procedure; her doctor kept reassuring her she wasn't pregnant), concerns about late abortions seem to fade.

Not surprisingly, the desire of anti-choice women to ensure most women become mothers by condemning any rejection of motherhood once a pregnancy has begun is accompanied by a different set of assumptions. Where pro-choice women assume the fetus is not * the same as a baby, anti-choice women assume that, in all important respects, it is just like a baby. While pro-choice women see the value of the fetus's life as a function of the quality of the life she can provide for it, anti-choice women think life, fetal or otherwise, is of irreducible and unequivocal value. Charlotte said: "I think that giving somebody a life is the best thing you can do for them."

The key to understanding women's assumptions regarding the value of fetal life is to remember that they *follow from* women's beliefs about the morality of abortion, they are not the reasons behind them. It is the belief about the place and position of motherhood in women's lives, in other words, that determines why some women favor abortion choice while others oppose it. When looked at this way, abortion provides the *means* for women to consider motherhood not as destiny, but as choice. For women who feel personally threatened by a society that makes motherhood a choice, making abortion a crime is merely the means through which society both restricts women's capacity to make this choice and voices its disapproval of it. For women who welcome the chance to choose motherhood, abortion is merely the tool necessary to bring about that choice. Whether or not a woman thinks having a choice about motherhood is a good thing will depend on a lot of factors, among them her social class and economic opportunities. It is hard for a woman to welcome the choice to be other than a mother if her financial situation prevents her from meaningfully exercising this choice.

• • •

But does re-casting the abortion debate as a conflict between women about motherhood actually solve any problems? Is it any less divisive for women to debate the value of motherhood than it has been for them to argue about the relative value of fetuses and women's rights to bodily autonomy? Is it really too risky for feminists to seriously challenge the amoral rights-based approach to abortion? How can the morality women have described be used to build consensus among a broad range of women who are both in favor of women's abortion freedom and concerned about abortion as a moral issue? In the next and final chapter, I try to answer some of these questions and point a way forward for pro-choice feminists as we enter the new millennium.

# · 6 ·

# Rights, Responsibilities, and Killing from Care

Pro-choice feminists have argued that abortion is a woman's issue, while anti-choice activists insist that it is a moral issue. In this book, I have put the case for returning abortion—as a moral issue—to women. Against feminists' descriptions of abortion as a simple medical procedure, and of the fetus as the "products of conception," I have established that women see abortion as a moral issue, and their fetuses as their highly valued could-be children. Against self-serving anti-choice claims to be the best representatives and only defenders of the fetus, I have shown pregnant women to act as moral agents in decisions about unplanned pregnancies, making the most responsible, caring, and appropriate decisions about the interconnected lives of themselves and the lives within them. I have demonstrated that in large part women assume they have the right to choose abortion and have become preoccupied with when, if ever, this choice is a moral one to make. I have suggested that we rename the abortion debate "the motherhood debate" so we remember that, in many ways, our interest in and anxieties about abortion reflect our interest in and anxiety over women's changing roles in the past century—their choices to be other than mothers.

It is the advent of high-tech fetal surveillance technologies and neo-natal care facilities on the one hand, and tactical miscalculations by the pro-choice movement on the other, that has led to the growing uncertainty of many in the pro-choice movement. According to bioethicist Daniel Callahan, director of the United States' Hastings Center, most people have two faces when it comes to abortion:

Most people seem to have a two-level response to the issue. One, on the surface is their public, professed position—what they tell strangers, poll-sters, and themselves when under attack. At another level, however, there is a more troubled private cauldron of jumbled beliefs, cross-cutting emo-tions and easily triggered raw-end sensibilities. I think of that as a kind of shadow self. That self is far less settled than the public self . . .[1]

In seeking to play down the moral dimensions of abortion, Calla-han argues, the pro-choice movement has not doused the fire sur-rounding the issue, but may only have fanned it:

The pro-choice movement . . . is particularly vulnerable to . . . medical and scientific developments. It has never made sufficient room in its public stance for a serious consideration of the fetus. Simultaneously, by deliber-ately cultivating a supposedly neutral, therapeutic language toward the medical act of abortion—calling it a procedure, a "termination of preg-nancy" and so on—it mistakenly seems to think it can pacify and comfort the secret self, minimizing and denaturing some unmistakable realities. There is still time to rectify that error, time for pro-choice adherents to show themselves as willing in practice as in theory to concede the moral un-certainty of abortion decisions. If this is not done, the combination of the new medical developments and too many secret selves for too long holding their doubts at bay may well begin shifting some public selves.[2]

The job of the pro-choice movement is to provide a moral de-fense of a woman's freedom to choose abortion, a defense that has women, not fetuses, at its center. A pro-choice abortion morality must be strongly feminist in nature, not an ethic of abstract princi-ples indiscriminately applied to the decontextualized lives of two-dimensional women. The problem with depersonalizing women and de-contextualizing their lives is that it gives the false impression that women—the way they make choices, and the choices they make—exist on a "level playing field." As a result, the ideal moral decision maker winds up looking an awful lot like a middle-class woman in her mid-twenties, sitting under a leafy green tree weigh-ing the pros and cons of motherhood and abortion. Daniel Callahan's prescription of the way women must negotiate the moral dilemma posed by unwanted pregnancy calls up an image of this ideal decision maker:

Even though the [abortion] choice should be the woman's, and . . . should be a private choice, it [is] still a serious moral choice. Once women had the choice it would then become important for them in their private lives to give thought to what could count as a morally justifiable choice . . . To be sure, the private moral wrestling would and could be a source of anguish and pain, but that is true of all critical moral choices, hardly unique to abortion . . . leave the choice to women but understand the choice to be a grave one, worthy of public no less than private reflection.[3]

We only have to remember the twelve-year-old girl in her twenty-sixth week of pregnancy by her mother's boyfriend to see the pernicious falsity of this vision. Women making decisions about motherhood and abortion are *not* on a level playing field. They are of different ages, have different financial resources and different amounts of education; they may have partners or be completely alone; they may be mentally incompetent, or physically abused. On the other hand, they may be educated, financially secure twenty-five-year-olds sitting under leafy green trees. Whatever the case, these factors will all impact on the timeliness and quality of the decision-making process women undergo when faced with an unwanted pregnancy. While women do and should treat abortion as a moral issue, their decision making and decisions will reflect not only their moral values but the complex social and financial realities of their lives. To forget this is both myopic and unfair. What we must do, says Rosalind Petchesky, is "reframe the moral arguments in a way that restores the dignity and centrality of women's moral judgment and locates the abortion decision within a woman's total situation."[4]

## Motherhood: Solving or Aggravating the Problem

The rancor of the abortion debate comes down to conflicting views of women's moral agency. Can women, should women, be trusted to make the best—the right—decisions about their pregnancies and motherhood, or should these decisions be made, or supervised, by others? Seen in this light, the abortion conflict can be understood as a power struggle between women on the one hand and those who would seek power over women's lives, bodies, and children on the other. What those on the anti-choice side seek is precisely the moral agency they are denying to women: the social power and the moral imprimatur to make decisions about when a woman will become a mother and how many children she will bear.

Some anti-choicers claim they seek this authority on behalf of God.[5] They claim that their faith commands them to do what is necessary to ensure that women lead "good Christian lives": lives in which childbearing and rearing are women's "privileged position and purpose in human history." An article by Paul Badham, the Chair of Church History and Senior Lecturer in Theology and Religious Studies at St. David's University College in the United Kingdom, questions the sincerity of such claims. While women have been having abortions since the dawn of recorded time, the first official peep from the Catholic church about the matter wasn't made until 1588, when Pope Sixtus V declared abortion to be murder. A mere three years later this opinion was reversed by his successor. Thus it wasn't until the middle of the nineteenth century (about the same time there was an upsurge in the popular advertising of abortion-inducing products and women's use of them) that Pope Pius IX decided that the embryo was a human being from conception and therefore that abortion was murder. Extensive research led Paul Badham to conclude that the church's absolutist stance on abortion "cannot legitimately find adequate justification by appeal to the Bible, Church tradition or Christian reasoning. Hence [anti-choice] pressure groups have no right to invoke the moral weight of historic Christianity for their opinions."[6]

It seems that what concerns church fathers about legal abortion is not much different from what worries other sorts of fathers: the erosion of their personal and institutional powers. It is well known that the Catholic church does little to stop women's relatively free access to abortions in many South American countries, yet stringently opposes making abortion services legal. Opposing abortion, explains Rosalind Petchesky, is a veiled way for some men to oppose the erosion of their control and power over women:

Men are not immune to the sense of personal loss and threat provoked by feminism and recent changes in the family and women's work . . . [anti-choice leader Paul] Weyrich . . . captures the essence of the . . . patriarchal *ressentiment:* "The fathers word has to prevail." With this unambiguous call to arms, he speaks not only as a New Right general but also as husband and father. And he speaks, too, as a leading patriarch in his church.[7]

American National Right to Life committee president J. C. Willke put things more baldly when he stated that pro-choice advocates "do violence to marriage by helping remove the right of a husband to protect the life of the child he has fathered in his wife's womb."[8]

The abortion issue is bound up with the reality of male privilege. Although the legal status of abortion has little impact on how many women seek and have abortions (though a large impact on how great a physical risk they bear in doing so), the anti-choice movement is undeterred in its quest to recriminalize the practice. The anti-choice agenda, in other words, is not to stop women having abortions so much as to ensure that abortion returns to being a "furtive, dangerous and necessarily degrading procedure."[9] It's hard for women to take charge of their reproductive lives, and thus their destinies, if they are classed as criminals, must be secretive about having an abortion, and are fearful of losing their lives, their health, or their fertility in unsafe procedures.

But it is not only men who feel threatened by the opportunities and freedom that abortion and feminism have made possible. Women make up the bulk of membership in the anti-choice movement (though not the majority of its leadership). This may seem contradictory. Why would women, who themselves may have had little choice about becoming mothers, fight to ensure that all other women—their daughters included—share the same fate? Perhaps one explanation is that anti-choice women fear that when women choose motherhood (as opposed to their being conscripted into it because they lack access to abortion), motherhood starts to look like "just" another job. If working mothers become the accepted norm, then women who are "just" mothers may start looking like dole-bludgers. "She's working *and* raising young children," the argument might go, "why are you *just* a mother?"

Another reason is the sad but frequently observed fact that women are often patriarchy's foot soldiers. It was women who bound their daughters' feet in China, and women in numerous Muslim countries today who bring their daughters to have their genitals mutilated. All too aware of the sanctions awaiting those who visibly defy the system that seeks to control them, these women mistakenly believe that things will be easier for themselves and their daughters if they do as they are told and don't make trouble.

## Speaking Out Honestly

If power and status—both men's and women's—are at the heart of the abortion issue, how will making these motivations more transparent in debates about motherhood reduce the friction surrounding the issue? To be honest, I'm not sure it will, but there are a few things that honesty might accomplish. First, sharing the language of motherhood means that at least pro- and anti-choicers are no longer talking apples (the right to control their bodies) and oranges (the right to life of fetuses). Not only does sharing the language of motherhood reduce terminological confusion, it reminds us that amidst considerable disagreements, women agree that abortion is a moral issue, and that the central value in the moral matrix is motherhood. Second, it means that what women are arguing about—motherhood—is not a cover story but what really makes them mad. There's little hope of solving a problem if you're not actually talking about the problem you need to solve. In addition, a shot of honesty into the arm of the abortion debate will reveal, once and for all, the hypocrisy of those who invoke God's will, or wave around bags of fetal parts in defense of their claims.

The truth is that straight and honest talk has been in short supply on both sides of the line. The hypocrisy of the anti-choice side has been matched by pro-choice attempts to quash the moral ambiguity around abortion with deceptive language or by ignoring the fetus. These tactics have not only been deceptive, they have failed. A *Newsweek* poll has found that 38 percent of Americans are unsure that their position on abortion is right, with 18 percent claiming that new scientific evidence about the early stages of fetal life had made them less approving than previously of abortion.[10] What this means is that even if many people's public positions on abortion remain static, the restlessness of many "secret selves" makes it impossible for the issue to be laid to rest. And so with each new technological advance, the issue can be driven into the open and re-hashed again.

Because the anti-choice movement has used feminist acknowledgment of the moral uncertainty of abortion as "proof" that abortion is wrong, feminists have grown reluctant to make such admissions. A similar debate about the wisdom of making certain admissions (irrespective of whether or not these admissions are true) has been taking place among academic feminists for years on the question of biological differences between men and women. The anti side argues that because such differences have been used successfully in the past by anti-feminists to oppress women, the only solution is to continue on the current course of denying such differences exist. The pros argue that even though male and female biological differences have been used to oppress women, discussing difference is not inherently oppressive. Male and female difference could also be used as grounds to privilege women, such as when it is argued that women are superior to men because they are more nurturing and caring. This turning of the tables—turning a "deficiency" into an "advantage"—is behind recent claims that women make better managers because they are less competitive and better team-players. The point is that "facts" may be used to support either side of an argument. Callahan underscores this point: "There has never been any straight line between . . . [facts] and the public argument about abortion. Various types of information lend themselves to varied moral, legal and political uses."[11] This means that while women's moral uncertainty about abortion can be used to undermine women's reproductive freedom, it can also be used to support it, as Sue O'Sullivan notes:

It's not as if the ambiguous or contradictory feelings women have about abortion have been imposed on them. Yet they are often taken as indications of an anti-abortion sentiment. A modern approach to abortion politics needs to allow women to have ambiguous feelings about abortion yet still be in favor of choice, still make the decision to have an abortion, and still support those who have abortions.[12]

So even if the long-term goal is to lay the abortion issue to rest so women can turn their energies to other things, the way to achieve that goal may be to open the issue right up: to explore women's experiences of both their rights and responsibilities in relation to abortion. In many ways, such an opening up is long overdue. Since the abortion "speak-outs" of the late 1960s and early 1970s, a whole generation of women has come of age. These women have enjoyed relatively free access to mostly safe and legal services, and at the same time have been bombarded with technological changes that have challenged prevailing views about the meaning and responsibility of pregnancy and the nature of fetal life. Many have heard a fetal heartbeat, seen a fetal ultrasound, and may even have given birth to a baby they'd already named because its sex was known from the amnio results. Feminists have been right to question what these advances have meant for women's understanding and experience of pregnancy and motherhood. Perhaps we also need to ask how such technologies have changed the ways women think about and experience abortion.

Once women have shared their experience, where do we go? From the inception of the women's movement, feminists have committed themselves to putting women's experiences at the center of their political theories and political actions; to making—to borrow a well-worn phrase—the personal the political. While traditionally this has meant seeing women's personal experiences as a consequence of social power, it can also mean using women's experiences as a jumping-off point for the development of feminist political theory on issues that matter to all women, like abortion. Where we can go, in other words, is toward a new feminist perspective on abortion that includes a thorough feminist discussion of the moral aspects of abortion.

Amending the pro-choice defense of abortion is not without its risks, of course. The pro- and anti-choice movements are huge, transnational entities that have spent years defining and refining their messages for public consumption. After so many years of public sparring, much of their organizational self-definitions and political rhetoric are reactions against the views and definitions of the other side. Who they are, in other words, is precisely what the other side is not. While the predictability of the political exchanges between the movements is mind-numbing for the observer, it reassures each side that they are not going to wind up without well-considered and pre-rehearsed rebuttals to the other's arguments; that they have the answers. Shifting abortion rhetoric could also topple the legal status quo, a situation feared by both sides as much as it is desired. While the middle-of-the-road nature of abortion laws and attitudes in the United States, Britain, and Australia makes neither the pro- nor the anti-choice movement happy, a slight shift to either side risks making at least one side that much more miserable.

Yet along with the risks and the uncertainties, there is the hope that if women are given the opportunity to relate their experiences of abortion over the last twenty-five years, an alternative defense of abortion can be structured. But first we must be clear about the moral code women are choosing to live by.

## The Moral Circle

What the women I have studied have described is a moral circle. Outside the circle is the athlete who becomes pregnant and has an abortion to improve her performance; women aborting an intended pregnancy to take up contest winnings of a trip overseas; and women who treat pregnancy and abortion, to use Janine's words, "lightly," as though "sweeping out some fluff, or some dirt." Admittedly, these examples are extreme. But just because few women would have such pregnancies or such abortions doesn't mean the consensus among women that they are wrong is unimportant. Rather, such abortions establish the outer limits of the moral circle, the boundary beyond which—the consensus position is—no woman should cross.

At this point, pro- and anti-choice views diverge. Because anti-choice and pro-choice women have fundamentally different views about the trustworthiness of other women, their assessments of which abortions fall within and outside the perimeter of the moral circle differ. For anti-choice women, almost all abortions—except perhaps those had by rape and incest victims and women whose own lives are at stake—would fall outside the circle. For pro-choice women, however, most women's abortions would remain inside the circle, although their placement in the area between the center and the outer edges might vary.

Once inside the circle, the moral focus of pro-choice women switches to the decision-making process of women choosing abortion. They hope and expect that each woman's abortion decision will be made thoughtfully, sorrowfully, and with respect for the sacredness of pregnancy and with love for their could-be child. That women's decisions will be, in other words, responsible ones to kill from care.

Inside the circle, trust—trust in women to act responsibly—is critical. What pro-choice women understood was that "killing from care" decisions often required life circumstances many women lacked: sufficient maturity; adequate time for reflection; emotional and financial stability; proximate and sympathetic medical care. The women I interviewed were also sensitive to the extraordinary complexity of the abortion decision (only the pregnant woman herself knows all one needs to know to make a good decision) and to the fact that it would be the pregnant woman above all who would "wear" whatever decision she made. So while there were expectations of women within the circle, there were few judgments.

This does not mean that pro-choice women abandoned morality when it came to the majority of women's abortion choices, but it does reveal both women's awareness of their own limitations to sit in judgment on others, and a respect for the judgment of other women. It is trust in the pregnant woman as a decision maker that was at the heart of these women's abortion morality. According to feminist ethicist Annette Baier, the very existence of a moral society is dependent on trust. The women I interviewed trusted that—within their means—pregnant women would do their utmost to treat the abortion decision as a moral one, and judge *themselves* accordingly.

The issue of self-judgment is an important one, because one of the fears feminists (rightly) have of acknowledging the moral aspects of abortion is that such acknowledgment risks women being called legally to account for mistaken choices they have made, perhaps by having their abortion "privileges" taken away. There is no logical connection between expressing moral doubts about a particular abortion decision and believing the law should punish those who fail to measure up morally, but that doesn't mean the anti-choice movement might not try to draw a connection in the public mind between the two. Moreover, convening panels to sit in judgment of women is fraught with problems. Who will sit on such a panel? Who will develop the standards against which women are judged? According to Lynda Birke, Susan Himmelweit, and Gail Vines, feminists must resist any calls to publicly judge or legally punish women who fail to pass moral muster because, first,

our . . . opinions should [not] be forced on others, any more than those of our opponents should. Second, [because] we cannot see any way to prevent such "bad" decisions being carried out, which do not have the danger of curtailing women's reproductive freedom in much more seriously harmful ways. And finally [because] we recognise that much greater harm can come of forcing women to bear children they do not want to bear than practically anything else; it is cruel both to the woman and to the child who would be born in such circumstances.[13]

## It's a Baby!

My mother and stepfather recently came over from the United States for a visit. This was the first time either had seen their youngest grandchild, an active, happy baby who likes to smile a lot. After an afternoon of beaming at Grandma and Grandpa and getting lots of cuddles in return, the baby was bundled off by my husband for a nap.

With just the adults around the table, the subject of this book came up. "It would be so much harder to have an abortion after you'd had one," my mother opined, nodding in the direction of the baby's room. "You know what you're doing. I mean, it's a *baby*!"

This took me aback. Remember, she was the one I was stuffing envelopes with for the pro-choice movement way back when and—to risk stating the obvious—she has been a mother herself.

'Yes," I said, "but that's precisely the reason you'd have an abortion—if you couldn't be in it body and soul. Because you know all that's involved. *Because* it's a *baby*."

My stepfather got it straightaway, but my mother was close behind. "That's true," she said, nodding her head slowly, "that's definitely true."

It is because our babies are so important—and in order that they remain so—that women must be given the legal right and be trusted with the moral responsibility to say about becoming a mother "yes," "not now," "not ever," or "not again." We must not forget how critical to our self-determination are our rights to choose. But neither can we ignore the pull of our secret selves toward a fuller picture of what abortion really means to us—as feminists and as responsible women.

# Appendix

## *Study Methodology*

The study was conducted to investigate the validity of Singer's and Wells's speculation about women's response to ectogenesis and to explore women's moral construction of abortion. The hypothesis was that women's construction of abortion would fundamentally differ from that articulated by severance theorists and that this would lead most women to reject ectogenesis as a moral solution to unwanted pregnancy. A further hypothesis was that women would consider the intentions and motivations of pregnant women who choose abortion to be a critical factor in their moral evaluation of the pregnant woman's choice. Forty-five Australian women were interviewed over a time period of five months. All the women were residents of the city of Melbourne, with the majority residing south of the central business district. Interviews were conducted after working hours either south of or within the central business district. Both the time and the locations were selected to allow working women to attend.

The project was advertised in a wide variety of media, and through relevant clubs, societies, and religious organizations. Advertisements read as follows:

### ABORTION AND TECHNOLOGY
### The Centre for Human Bioethics

Women are needed to participate in group interviews on the topic of current abortion practices and upcoming medical developments in this area. Participants will be asked what they believe women's intentions are when they abort, and for their responses to new neo-natal technology. The research is the thesis component of a Master of Bioethics.

All women of childbearing age are welcome. You do not need to have had an abortion or be an "expert" on any of the issues. All viewpoints on the abortion issues are welcome. All information and the identity of participants will be kept in the strictest of confidence.

Your involvement would be greatly appreciated, and all efforts will be made to arrange times and places suited to your busy schedule. Please contact Leslie Cannold during day or evening hours for further information.

When women who were interested contacted the researcher through the telephone number supplied in the advertisement, an interview appointment was arranged. An attempt was made to place women in groups with other women with similar attitudes toward abortion, and this was mostly, though not always, successful. Because some difficulty arose in assembling the sample of women opposed to abortion rights, women in this group who did make contact were encouraged to bring friends along to the interview, which several of them did. The only criterion for exclusion was age, with the sample restricted to women who identified themselves to be of childbearing age.

Interviews lasted anywhere between one half hour to two and one half hours. In general, interview sessions with women opposed to abortion rights tended to be of shorter duration than those with women in favor of abortion rights. Prior to the interview, explanatory or plain language statements were provided to participants, and signatures on consent forms sought. Women were given the explanatory statement, with the name and contact information of the researcher, and a copy of their signed consent form to keep. A questionnaire was administered to collect demographic information and abortion history and views. Specifically, women were asked their age, their position on abortion, the highest educational qualification they had obtained, their marital status, whether or not they had children and if they did, how many, whether or not they were a full-time homemaker, and whether they had ever had an abortion. Women were invited to provide their address to the researcher if they wished to be notified of details of any publications. At the conclusion of the interview, women were "debriefed," or given the opportunity to hear more about the rationale of the study and the working hypotheses.

## PROFILE OF PARTICIPATING WOMEN

From the questionnaire, the following picture of the sample emerges. Of the forty-five women interviewed, twelve women (27 percent) described themselves as "opposed to abortion in all circumstances—no exceptions"; nine women (20 percent) described themselves as "opposed to abortion in most circumstances—a few exceptions where in favour"; nine women (20 percent) said they were "in favour of abortion rights in most circumstances—a few exceptions where not in favour"; and fifteen women (33 percent) said they were "totally in favour of abortion rights—no exceptions." None of the women said they were "undecided/indifferent" to the issue.

For purposes of analyses, the categories "opposed to abortion in all circumstances—no exceptions" and "opposed to abortion in most circumstances—a few exceptions where in favour" were compressed into a single category renamed "women opposed to abortion rights." Similarly the two categories expressing partial or complete support of abortion rights were compressed into a single category renamed "women in favour of abortion rights." Utilizing these two categories we discover the following:

### Age

The ages of participants ranged between 19 and 53, with the bulk of the women between the ages of 20 and 40. Eighteen percent of the women were 20 years old or younger, 39 percent of the women were between age 21 and 30, 27 percent of the women were between 31 and 40 years of age, and 18 percent of the women interviewed were aged 40 or over. Of the women opposed to abortion, 33 percent were 20 years old or younger, 29 percent between the ages of 21 and 30 with the remaining 38 percent of the sample divided evenly between the 31 to 40 age group, and the over 40s. On the other hand, only 4 percent of women in favor of abortion rights were 20 years old or younger, with 46 percent of this sub-sample between the ages of 21 and 30. Thirty-three percent of women in this group were between the ages of 31 and 40, with 17 percent over 40 years old. To summarize these results, we see that the bulk (62 percent) of women opposed to abortion rights were aged 30 or under, with most (79 percent) of women in favor of abortion rights between the ages of 21 and 40.

## Education

Women who left school in tenth grade (a formal option in Australia) comprised 15.6 percent of the sample, with women who had completed high school making up the largest group with 33.3 percent. Those holding post-graduate diplomas made up 17.8 percent of the sample, while those with undergraduate university degrees comprised 20 percent. In the sample, 13.3 percent of the women held post-graduate degrees. The bulk of women opposed to abortion rights had either left school prior to receiving their diploma (24 percent) or their diploma constituted their highest educational qualification (48 percent). No women in this group held a post-graduate qualification. On the other hand, only 8.3 percent of women in favor of abortion rights left school prior to graduation, with the rest of this sub-sample falling more or less evenly into the other educational categories. This finding is consistent with other work in this area, which indicates that higher education levels are correlated with more liberal attitudes toward abortion.[1]

## Marital Status

Married and single women made up equal percentages of the sample (47 percent), with 6 percent of the women describing themselves as divorced. The 6 percent of the sample that described themselves as divorced were made up entirely of women in favor of abortion rights.

## Children

Just over half the sample were childless. Thirteen percent had one child, 13 percent had two children, 9 percent had three children, and 11 percent had four children or more. There were no discernable trends among women in favor of abortion rights and women opposed to abortion rights in this category.

*Work Status*
Sixty-four percent of the women currently worked outside of the home, while 36 percent described themselves as homemakers. Fifty-seven percent of women opposed to abortion rights worked outside the home, as compared to 43 percent of this group that were homemakers. In contrast, fully 71 percent of women in favor of abortion rights worked outside the home, with only 29 percent describing themselves as homemakers. Again, this finding is consistent with other work in the area that suggests there is a positive correlation between employment status and more liberal attitudes toward abortion.[2]

*Income*
The largest proportion of women in the sample lived in households where the income was $20,000 or less. Households of $36,000– $50,000 and $21,000–$35,000 comprised the next largest groups, with only 7 percent from households earning between $51,000 and $75,000 and just 9 percent of women coming from households with incomes over $76,000. No trends could be identified by comparing income distribution of women opposed to abortion rights with women in favor of abortion rights.

*Abortion History*
Almost one-third of the women (31 percent) had undergone an abortion. Of the women opposed to abortion rights, only one (4.8 percent) had undergone a termination, while for women in favor of abortion rights, over half (54 percent) had abortion in their history.

INTERVIEW QUESTIONS

Women were asked four questions, always in the same order. Nondirective questioning techniques were used to facilitate discussion of the issues. The questions were as follows:

1. If pregnant with a child you could not keep, would you choose

to have an abortion, or would you choose to have the child and give it up for adoption? Why?

2. Imagine that you are two months pregnant. You do not want to raise the child or are unable to do so and thus must decide between having an abortion or carrying the child to term and giving it up for adoption. As you are considering these options, a doctor approaches you and tells you that you have a third option. Thanks to technology, it is now possible for you to abort your fetus without killing it. Your fetus can be extracted from your body and transferred to an artificial womb where it will be grown until it is able to live outside of that artificial womb. At around nine months, it will then be put up for adoption. The doctor informs you that this procedure carries no more medical risks or inconvenience to you than the traditional abortion method.[3] Would you chose this third option?

3. Imagine that your relative suffers from a disease that can be successfully treated with fetal tissue. Up to now, your relative has used tissue available from abortions that were not done with the intention of providing tissue for this use. Lately, however, not enough abortions have been done to cope with the increasing demand for tissue, and your relative has requested that you become pregnant in order to abort the fetus to assist in her treatment. Do you do it?

4. Imagine that you have become pregnant voluntarily. Just as you begin to show, you discover you have won an all expenses paid trip for two to Barcelona for the Olympics. However, for promotional reasons, the people offering you the trip don't want you to look pregnant. They say that you must have an abortion in order to take up the winnings, which because they revolve around the Olympics, can not be delayed until after the child is born. What would you do?

The intent of the questions was to discover the women's position on abortion (questions 1–4), the way they justified these positions (questions 1–4), their response to ectogenesis and the relationship between this response and their position on abortion (question 2), and the moral framework supporting their position on abortion (questions 3–4).

A few remarks about some of the questions are necessary. In question 1, the intention was to pursue why women choose either abortion or adoption, not their reasons for being unable to keep the child. Thus, for example, if a woman would state her preference for abortion in terms of her inability to financially support a child, she would be asked why she chose abortion rather than adoption as a remedy to this problem.

In a number of interview sessions, issues and concerns were raised about the role of men in a society where ectogenesis was available. Most prominent of these were questions regarding the meaning of the male genetic contribution to the fetus in a world where conception, gestation, and birth could be separated. These issues were pursued and are reported on in the main text.

Finally, in one of the early sessions with women in favor of abortion rights, a woman raised a moral dilemma analogous to the one described in question 4. She presented the case of a female athlete who became pregnant to utilize the hormone change that accompanies pregnancy to assist her athletic performance, and then she procured an abortion before the pregnancy came to term. This dilemma was raised and discussed by the interviewer with women in a number of subsequent sessions.

# Notes

## Epigraphs (p. vii)

1. R. Petchesky, *Abortion and Woman's Choice: The State, Sexuality, and Reproductive Freedom* (Boston: Northeastern University Press), 1985, p. 341.

2. C. Gilligan, *In a Different Voice: Psychological Theory and Women's Development* (Cambridge and London: Harvard University Press, 1982), p. 116.

3. C. Mackenzie, "Abortion and embodiment" in *Troubled Bodies: Critical Perspectives on Postmodernism, Medical Ethics, and the Body*, ed. P. Komesaroff (Melbourne: Melbourne University Press, 1995), p. 43.

4. S. Kitzinger, *Ourselves as Mothers: The Universal Experience of Motherhood* (London, Ontario, Moorebank, NSW, Aukland: Doubleday, 1992), p. viii.

## Introduction to the American Edition (pp. xiv–xxv)

1. Personal communication.

2. C. M. Condit, *Decoding Abortion Rhetoric: Communicating Social Change* (Champaign: University of Illinois Press, 1990); D. M. Condit, "Fetal personhood: political identity under construction," *Expecting Trouble: Surrogacy, Fetal Abuse and New Reproductive Technologies*, ed. P. Boling (Boulder, Colo.: Westview Press, 1995); R. Petchesky, "Foetal images: the power of visual culture in the politics of reproduction," *Reproductive Technologies, Gender, Motherhood and Medicine*, ed. M. Stanworth (U.K.: Polity Press, 1987), pp. 57–80.

3. V. Hartouni, *Cultural Conceptions: On Reproductive Technologies and the Remaking of Life* (Minneapolis and London: University of Minnesota Press, 1997).

4. K. Newman, *Fetal Positions: Individualism, Science, Visuality* (Stanford: Stanford University Press, 1996).

5. K. Luker, *Abortion and the Politics of Motherhood* (Berkeley: University of California Press, 1984).

6. F. Ginsburg, *Contested Lives: The Abortion Debate in an American Community* (Berkeley: University of California Press, 1989).

7. P. Gomberg, "Abortion and the morality of nurturance," *Canadian Journal of Philosophy* 21, no. 4 (1991): 513–24.

8. L. Cannold, P. Singer, H. Kuhse, L. Gruen, "What is the justice-care debate *really* about?" *Midwest Studies in Philosophy* 20 (1996): 357–77.

9. See, for example, N. Hartsock and S. Harding, "The feminist stand-point: developing the ground for a specifically feminist historical material-ism," *Discovering Reality: Feminist Perspective on Epistemology, Meta-physics, Methodology, and the Philosophy of Science,* ed. S. Harding and M. Hintikka (Dordrecht: Reidel, 1983).

10. Foucault as quoted in S. Hekman, "Truth and method: feminist standpoint theory revisited," *Signs* 22, no. 2 (1997): 345.

11. V. Held, *Feminist Morality: Transforming Culture, Society, and Politics* (Chicago and London: University of Chicago Press, 1993); and P. Lauritzen, "Hear no evil, see no evil, think no evil: ethics and the appeal to experience," *Hypatia* 12, no. 2 (1997): 83–104.

12. *Reproductive Freedom News,* 1998.

13. Ibid.

14. Ibid., 1996.

15. S. Watkins, "'Cavalier' abortionists slated by pro-life," *The Age* (Melbourne), 27 April 1998, p.6.

16. *Reproductive Freedom News,* 1996.

17. I am not the first to recognize this danger. See, for example, N. Rhoden, "Trimesters and technology: revamping *Roe v. Wade*," *Yale Law Journal* 95 (1986): 639–97.

18. N. Boyce, "Off the wall: wild ideas in medicine find a willing sponsor," *New Scientist* (1998), 11 April 1998, p. 13.

19. AAP, "Womb donor hope," *The Age* (Melbourne), 25 May 1998, p. 3.

## Introduction to the Australian Edition (pp. xxvii–xxxii)

1. J. Smith, "Abortion and moral development theory: listening with different ears," *International Philosophical Quarterly* 28, no. 109 (March 1988): 31–51.

2. K. Kissane, "Abortion doubts redefine debate," *The Age,* 25 October 1995, p. 19.

3. E. Fairweather, "Abortion: The Feelings Behind the Slogans" in *Women's Health: A Spare Rib Reader,* ed. S. O'Sullivan (London: Pandora, 1987), pp. 199–200.

4. I am grateful to Dr. Michael Smith, who came up with the phrase "Killing from care" during a casual conversation with me about my research findings.

5. M. Claire, *The Abortion Dilemma: Personal Views on a Public Issue* (New York: Insight Books, Plenum Press, 1995), pp. 19–20.

6. *Ms.* 7, no. 3 (November/December 1996): 27.

7. Dr. Margie Ripper of the Women's Studies Department at the University of Adelaide was the first person to pose a version of this rhetorical question.

## Chapter 1. Is It Right? (pp. 1–16)

1. S. Faludi, *Backlash: The Undeclared War against Women* (London: Vintage, 1992), p. 451.

2. While some neonatologists seem to feel that the mere survival of a very young fetus is an accomplishment, others have concerns about the high percentage of extremely low-birthweight infant who suffer some form of physical, psychological, social, and/or intellectual disablement as a result of their extreme prematurity. See S. W. Teplin et al. "Neurodevelopmental health and growth status at age 6 years of children with birth weights less than 1001 grams," in *The Journal of Pediatrics* 118 (1991): 768–77. Also Saigal et al., "Cognitive abilities and school performance of extremely low birth weight children and matched term control children at age 8 years: A regional study," in *The Journal of Pediatrics* 118 (1991): 751–60.

3. P. Singer and D. Wells, *The Reproduction Revolution: New Ways of Making Babies* (Oxford: Oxford University Press, 1984; published in the United States as *Making Babies*), p. 135.

4. Ibid.

5. C. Bertoia and J. Drakich, "The fathers' rights movement," *Journal of Family Issues* 14, no. 4 (1993): 592–615; quote on p. 593. See also R. Graycar, "Equal rights versus fathers' rights: the child custody debate in Australia," and N. Holstrust, S. Sevenhuijsen, and A. Verbraken, "Rights for fathers and the state: recent developments in custody politics in the Netherlands," in *Child Custody and the Politics of Gender*, ed. C. Smart and S. Sevenhuijsen (London: Routledge, 1989), pp. 158–89 and pp. 51–76.

6. Bertoia and Drakich, "The fathers' rights movement," p. 603.

7. Ibid., p. 607.

8. Ibid., p. 613.

9. K. McDonnell, *Not an Easy Choice: A Feminist Re-examines Abortion* (Boston: South End Press, 1984).

10. J. J. Thomson, "A defence of abortion," in *Applied Ethics*, ed. P. Singer (Oxford: Oxford University Press, 1986).

11. C. Overall, *Ethics and Human Reproduction: A Feminist Analysis* (Boston: Allen & Unwin, 1987).

12. K. Lucker, *Abortion and the Decision Not to Contracept* (Berkeley: University of California Press, 1975); *Abortion and the Politics of Motherhood* (Berkeley: University of California Press, 1984). Other published and well-regarded studies that have focused on women's experience of abortion are: L. Francke, *The Ambivalence of Abortion* (New York: Random House, 1978); C. Gilligan, *In a Different Voice: Psychological Theory and Women's Development* (Cambridge: Harvard University Press, 1982); F. Ginsburg, *Contested Lives: The Abortion Debate in an American Community* (Berkeley: University of California Press, 1989); K. Luker, *Abortion and the Politics of Motherhood* (Berkeley: University of California Press, 1984); A. Neustatter and G. Newson, *Mixed Feelings: The Experience of Abortion* (Sydney: Pluto Press, 1986); L. Ryan, M. Ripper, and B. Buttfield, *We Women Decide: Women's Experience of Seeking Abortion in Queensland, South Australia and Tasmania 1985–1992* (South Australia: Flinders University Women's Social Studies Unit, Faculty of Social Sciences, 1994); and M. Zimmerman, *Passage Through Abortion* (New York: Praegar Special Studies, 1977).

13. K. Luker, *Abortion and the Decision Not to Contracept.*

14. Greater detail about the study can be found in L. Cannold, "Women, ectogenesis and ethical theory," *Journal of Applied Philosophy* 12, no. 1 (1995): 57–64.

15. Personal communication.

16. J. Davies, "New push on abortion pill," *The Age,* 18 May 1997, p. 1.

17. J. Lynxwiler and D. Gay, "Reconsidering race differences in abortion attitudes," *Social Science Quarterly* 75, no. 1 (1994): 67–84.

18. J. Lazzaro and J. Waugh, *Abortion, An Act of Love: Sixteen Women Tell Their Stories* (Melbourne: Melbourne University Social Enquiry and Social Work Research Project (1991), p. 44.

19. Gilligan, *In a Different Voice,* p. 21.

20. Ginsburg, *Contested Lives,* p. 149.

21. Personal communication.

## Chapter 2. The Way It Is Now (pp. 18–44)

1. P. Horsley and S. Tremellin, eds., "Old fights and new challenges: a roundtable discussion on abortion," *Healthsharing Women* 6, nos. 6–7 (June–September 1996): 15.

2. NHMRC, "Services for the termination of pregnancy in Australia: a review," draft consultation document, September 1995, pp. 11–16; NHMRC, "An information paper on termination of pregnancy in Australia," Commonwealth of Australia, 1996, p. 7.

3. A. Matheson, "The abortion scam: pro-life's shocking new tactics," *New Woman,* April 1996, p. 76.

4. Personal communication.

5. R. Petchesky, "Foetal images: the power of visual culture in the politics of reproduction," in *Reproductive Technologies: Gender, Motherhood and Medicine,* ed. M. Stanworth (Minneapolis: University of Minnesota Polity Press, 1987), p. 58.

6. J. Hadley, *Abortion: Between Freedom and Necessity* (London: Vintage, 1996), p. 32.

7. Personal communication.

8. NHMRC, "Services for the termination of pregnancy," pp. 35–36; NHMRC, "An information paper on termination of pregnancy in Australia," p. 49.

9. Ryan, Ripper and Buttfield, *We Women Decide,* p. 66.

10. Ibid., p. 203.

11. E. Fairweather, "Abortion: the feelings behind the slogans," p. 199.

12. L. R. Churchill and J. J. Siman, "Abortion and the rhetoric of individual rights," *The Hastings Center Report* 12, no. 1 (February 1982): 9–12.

13. R. Dworkin as quoted in ibid., p. 10.

14. Ibid., p. 11.

15. Hadley, *Abortion: Between Freedom and Necessity,* p. 73.

16. C. Smart, *Feminism and the Power of Law* (London: Routledge, 1989), p. 143.

17. Ibid, p. 153.

18. Petchesky, "Foetal images," p. 79.

19. Hadley, *Abortion: Between Freedom and Necessity*, p. 194.

20. L. Birke, S. Himmelweit, and G. Vines, *Tomorrow's Child: Reproductive Technologies in the 90s* (London: Virago, 1990), p. 289.

21. R. Dunne, "Dissenting views 1," *Surrogacy: Report 1*, The National Bioethics Consultative Committee, Commonwealth of Australia, 1990, p. 47.

22. Hadley, *Abortion: Between Freedom and Necessity*, p. 52.

23. Claire, *The Abortion Dilemma*, p. 245.

24. J. Finlay, "A fatal concern," *The Age*, 2 November 1996, p. 16. In response to L. Cannold, "Killing from care: a woman's sorrow," *The Age*, 1 November 1996, p. 23.

25. Fairweather, "Abortion: the feelings behind the slogans," p. 196.

26. C. Vinzant, "The ghastly inside story of how the right-to-life movement stockpiles and uses aborted fetuses," *Spy*, May 1993, p. 65.

27. Ibid., p. 60.

28. Hadley, *Abortion: Between Freedom and Necessity*, p. 55.

29. Petchesky, "Foetal images," p. 57.

30. B. K. Rothman, *The Tentative Pregnancy: Pre-natal Diagnosis and the Future for Motherhood* (New York: Viking, 1986), p. 114.

31. Petchesky, "Foetal images," p. 63.

32. A. Oakley, "From walking wombs to test-tube babies," in Stanworth, ed., *Reproductive Technologies*, p. 42.

33. C. M. Condit, *Decoding Abortion Rhetoric: Communicating Social Change* (Champaign: University of Illinois Press, 1990), p. 82.

34. Ibid., p. 83.

35. Ibid., p. 85.

36. D. M. Condit, "Fetal personhood: political identity under construction," in *Expecting Trouble: Surrogacy, Fetal Abuse and New Reproductive Technologies*, ed. P. Boling (Boulder: Westview Press, 1995), p. 31.

37. N. Wolf, "Our bodies, our souls: rethinking pro-choice rhetoric," *The New Republic*, 16 October 1995, p. 34.

38. J. Lazzaro and J. Waugh, et al., *Abortion, an Act of Love: Sixteen Women Tell Their Stories* (Melbourne: Melbourne University, 1991), p. 78.

39. Claire, *The Abortion Dilemma*, p. 73.

40. Wolf, "Our bodies, our souls," p. 28.

41. Personal communication.

42. R. Albury, "Contesting technology, representing women: hard questions about activism," unpublished manuscript, n.d., p. 14.

43. Birke, Himmelweit, and Vines, *Tomorrow's Child*, p. 25.

44. Horsley, Tremelin, eds., "Old fights and new challenges," p. 14.

45. L. Cannold, "A major step for abortion rights," *Healthsharing Women* 5, no. 1 (August–September 1994): 4.

46. L. Cannold, "The ongoing debate about RU 486," *Healthsharing*

*Women* 5, no. 2 (October–November 1994), pp. 3–8. Also L. Cannold, "Abortion pill hope," *The Age*, 31 May 1994, p. A18.

47. R. Petchesky, "Abortion in the 1980s: feminist morality and women's health" in *Women, Health and Healing: Toward a New Perspective*, ed. E. Levin and V. Olesen (New York: Tavistock, 1985), p. 43.

## Chapter 3. The Downward Spiral of Viability and the Urgent Need for Change (47–70)

1. "South Carolina high court reinstates conviction for mother's behavior during pregnancy," *Reproductive Freedom News* 13, 26 July 1996, p. 4.

2. "Florida Appeals Court allows prosecution of pregnant woman who shot herself," *Reproductive Freedom News* 5, 5 April 1996, p. 3. Also Claire, *The Abortion Dilemma*, p. 257.

3. L. Cannold-McDonald, "Technical victory, political defeat," *The Age*, 8 July 1992, p. 16.

4. Hadley, *Abortion: Between Freedom and Necessity*, p. 11.

5. Center for Reproductive Law & Policy, "The status of a woman's right to choose abortion," *Reproductive Freedom in the States*, 1995, p. 2.

6. D. M. Condit, "Fetal personhood," p. 41.

7. Oakley, "From walking wombs to test-tube babies," p. 51.

8. L. Purdy, "The baby in the body," *The Hastings Center Report* 24, no. 1 (1994): 31–32.

9. T. Elkins, H. F. Andersen, et al., "Court-ordered cesarean section: an analysis of ethical concerns in compelling cases," *American Journal of Obstetrics and Gynecology* 161, no. 1 (1989): 150–54.

10. I. M. Bernstein, M. Watson, et al., "Maternal brain death and prolonged fetal survival," *Obstetrics & Gynecology* 74, no. 3, pt. 2 (1989): 434–37.

11. Purdy, "The baby in the body," p. 32.

12. Dworkin as quoted in Oakley, "From walking wombs to test-tube babies," p. 55.

13. C. Overall, *Ethics and Human Reproduction: A feminist analysis* (Boston: Allen & Unwin, 1987), p. 55.

14. D. M. Condit "Fetal personhood," p. 39 and K. Pollitt, "Fetal rights: a new assault on feminism," *The Nation*, 26 March 1990, p. 409.

15. Pollitt, "Fetal rights," pp. 409–18.

16. D. M. Condit, "Fetal personhood," p. 39.

17. V. Kolder, J. Gallagher, and M. Parsons, "Court-ordered obstetrical interventions," *The New England Journal of Medicine* 316, no. 19 (7 May 1987): pp. 1192–96.

18. M. Wallace, *Health Care and the Law: A Guide for Nurses* (North Ryde, N.S.W.: The Law Book Company 1991), p. 62.

19. L. Cannold, "'There is no evidence to suggest': changing the way we judge information for disclosure in the informed consent process," *Hypatia* 12, no. 2 (1997).

20. D. M. Condit, "Fetal personhood," p. 42.

21. B. Jordan, *Birth in Four Cultures: A Crosscultural Investigation of Childbirth in Yucatan, Holland, Sweden, and the United States,* fourth edition (Prospect Heights, Illinois: Waveland Press, 1993), p. 149.

22. Ibid.

23. Oakley, "From walking wombs to test-tube babies," p. 44.

24. S. Brown, J. Lumley, R. Small, and J. Astbury, *Missing Voices: the Experience of Motherhood* (Melbourne: Oxford University Press, 1994), p. 34.

25. Petchesky, "Foetal images," p. 66.

26. Pollitt, "Fetal rights," p. 414.

27. Evolutionary biologist Dr. David Haig as quoted in M. Lipsitch, "The battle before birth," *The Age,* 9 August 1993, p. 3.

28. Petchesky, "Foetal images," p. 60.

29. C. M. Condit, *Decoding Abortion Rhetoric,* p. 87.

30. D. Concar, "Into the mind of the unborn," *New Scientist,* 19 October 1996, pp. 40–45.

31. Petchesky, "Foetal images," p. 61.

32. C. M. Condit, *Decoding Abortion Rhetoric,* p. 86.

33. D. M. Condit, "Fetal personhood," p. 35.

34. I. Young, "Pregnant embodiment: subjectivity and alienation," *The Journal of Medicine and Philosophy* 9, (1984): 45.

35. P. Debelle, "Ethics in embryo," *Good Weekend Magazine,* 6 April 1991, pp. 18–22.

36. D. Grundmann, "Abortion after twenty weeks in clinical practice: practical, ethical and legal issues" in *The Proceedings of the Conference: Ethical Issues in Prenatal Diagnosis and the Termination of Pregnancy,* ed. J. McKie (Melbourne: Monash University Centre for Human Bioethics, 1994).

37. Hadley, *Abortion: Between Freedom and Necessity,* p. 68.

38. NHMRC, "Services for the termination of pregnancy," p. 58.

39. Ryan, Ripper, and Buttfield, *We Women Decide,* p. 102.

40. Two New York nurses recently lost their jobs because of their refusal to perform abortions. Center for Reproductive Law and Policy, "New York judge says dismissed anti-abortion nurses cannot sue hospital," *Reproductive Freedom News* 13, 18 July 1997, p. 5.

41. D. Krutli, "Mid-trimester abortion service within a public hospital," *Women and Surgery: Conference Proceedings* (Melbourne: Healthsharing Women, 1990), p. 103.

42. Claire, *The Abortion Dilemma,* p. 121.

43. NHMRC, "Services for the termination of pregnancy," pp. 22–23.

44. P. Singer and H. Kuhse, *Should the Baby Live?: The Problem of Handicapped Infants* (Oxford: Oxford University Press, 1985), p. 151.

45. Rance v. Mid-Downs Health Authority & Storr, *Australian Health and Medical Law Reporter,* Clinical Practice, pars. 21–740, p. 24902.

46. R. Rowland, *Living Laboratories: Women and Reproductive Technologies* (Sydney: Pan Macmillan, 1993, p. 46.

47. Ibid., p. 77.

48. S. Dow, "Technology of hope poses new dilemmas," *The Age,* 25 July 1996, A13.

49. T. Ewing, "IVF breakthrough hailed," *The Age,* 2 May 1997, p. 1.

50. S. Dow, "Technology of hope poses new dilemmas," *The Age,* A13.

51. Dr. Neil Campbell, personal communication, 25 July 1996.

52. C. Bulletti et al., "Early human pregnancy in vitro utilizing an artificially perfused uterus," *Fertility and Sterility* 49, no. 6 (1988): 991.

53. P. Hadfield, "Japanese pioneers raise kid in rubber womb," *New Scientist,* 25 April 1992, p. 5.

## Chapter 4. Pregnancy (pp. 73–96)

1. J. G. Thornton, H. M. McNamara, and I. A. Montague, "Would you rather be a "birth" or a "genetic" mother? If so, how much?," *Journal of Medical Ethics* 20, no. 2, 1994, pp. 87–92.

2. R. Dunne, "Dissenting views," p. 49.

3. N. Lowinsky, *The Motherline: Every Woman's Journey to Find Her Female Roots* (New York: Putnam's, 1992), p. 14.

4. Mead as discussed in Oakley, "From walking wombs to test-tube babies," p. 53.

5. M. Stanworth, "Reproductive technologies and the deconstruction of motherhood," in *Reproductive Technologies: Gender, Motherhood and Medicine* (Minneapolis: University of Minnesota Press, 1987), p. 16.

6. Quoted in Oakley, "From walking wombs to test-tube babies," p. 55.

7. E. Kane, *Birth Mother* (Sydney: Sun Books, 1990), p. xvii.

8. Ibid., p. xxii.

9. NHMRC, "Services for the termination of pregnancy," p. 42, and A. Kulczycki, M. Potts, and A. Rosenfield, "Abortion and fertility regulation," *The Lancet* 347 (1996): 1663–68.

10. C. AbouZahr, "The epidemiology of unsafe abortion," *The Kangaroo,* December 1994, p. 164.

11. S. Henshaw and K. Kost, "Abortion, patients in 1994–1995: characteristics and contraceptive use," *Family Planning Perspectives* 28, no. 4 (1996): 1–16.

12. M. Zimmerman, *Passage Through Abortion: The Personal and Social Reality of Women's Experience* (New York: Praeger Special Studies, 1977), p. 77.

13. Francke, *The Ambivalence of Abortion,* p. 39.

14. S. Powell and H. Stagoll, *When You Can't Have a Child* (North Sydney: Drummond: Allen & Unwin, 1992), p. 5. Also Rowland, *Living Laboratories,* p. 47.

15. Rowland, *Living Laboratories,* p. 52.

16. L. Cannold, "The new progestogen 'third generation' oral contraceptive pills: how safe are they?," *Healthsharing Women* 6, nos. 3–4 (1996): 14–18.

17. K. Hicks, *Surviving the Dalkon Shield IUD: Women v. the Pharmaceutical Industry* (New York and London: Teachers College Press, 1994).

18. Luker, *Abortion and the Decision Not to Contracept,* p. 16.

19. Ibid., p. 20.

20. Ibid., p. 35.

21. Ibid., p. 27.

22. Ibid., p. 27.

23. Ibid., p. 65.

24. D. Handelsman, "Male contraception: present and future," *On the Level* 4, no. 2 (1996): 13.

25. J. Bruce, "Reproductive choice: the responsibilities of men and women," *On the Level* 4, no. 2 (1996): 6.

26. Zimmerman, *Passage Through Abortion,* p. 106.

27. A. Clissa, "Unplanned pregnancy," *On the Level* 4, no. 2 (1996): 30.

28. Francke, *The Ambivalence of Abortion,* p. 39.

29. Zimmerman, *Passage Through Abortion,* p. 88.

30. E. Bowtell, "Condoms, coitus and adolescents," *On the Level* 4, no. 2 (1996): 17.

31. W. Marsiglio, "Husbands sex-role preferences and contraceptive intentions: the case of the male pill," *Sex Roles* 12, nos. 5–6 (1985): 661.

32. Bowtell, "Condoms, coitus and adolescents," p. 16.

33. Kitzinger, *Ourselves as Mothers,* p. 74.

34. A. Eisenberg, H. Murkoff, and S. Hathaway, *What to Expect When You're Expecting* (Sydney, Aukland: Angus & Robertson, 1993), p. xx.

35. Kitzinger, *Ourselves as Mothers,* p. 79.

36. Brown, Lumley et al., *Missing Voices,* pp. 31–49.

37. M. Crouch and L. Manderson, *New Motherhood: Cultural and Personal Transitions in the 1980s* (Amsterdam: Gordon and Breach, 1993), p. 7.

38. The Boston Women's Health Collective, *The New Our Bodies, Ourselves* (New York: Simon & Schuster, 1984), p. 343.

39. M. Merleau-Ponty, *The Phenomenology of Perception,* trans. Colin Smith (New York: Humanities Press, 1962), p. 82.

40. The term "man-made language" was coined by Dale Spender. D. Spender, *Man Made Language* (London: Routledge & Kegan Paul, 1985).

41. Young, "Pregnant embodiment," p. 45.

42. R. M. Polatnick, "Diversity in women's liberation ideology: how a black and a white group of the 1960s viewed motherhood," *Signs* 21, no. 3 (1996): 683.

43. K. Kennison and K. Hirsch, *Mothers: Twenty Stories of Contemporary Motherhood* (New York: North Point Press, 1996), p. 5.

44. Lowinsky, *The Motherline,* pp. 39–40.

45. Dunn, "Dissenting Views 1," p. 49.

46. A. Rich, *Of Woman Born* (New York: W. W. Norton, 1976), pp. 47–48.

47. Regis Dunne, "Dissenting Views," p. 49.

48. S. Ross, "Abortion and the death of the fetus," *Philosophy & Public Affairs* 2, no. 3 (1982): 236.

49. Hadley, *Abortion: Between Freedom and Necessity,* p. 18.

50. N. Wolf, "Staking a right to struggle," *The Age,* 25 October 1995, p. 19.

## Chapter 5. The Good Mother (pp. 98–122)

1. E. Karlin, "An abortionist's credo," *Sunday New York Times,* 19 March 1995, p. 32.

2. S. Brownmiller, *Femininity* (New York: Fawcett Columbine, 1984), p. 214.

3. B. Wearing, *The Ideology of Motherhood: A Study of Sydney Suburban Mothers* (Sydney: Allen & Unwin, 1984), p. 48.

4. Brown, Lumley et al., *Missing Voices,* p. 151.

5. Ibid., p. 160.

6. S. Heath, "Marriage, motherhood and other mayhem," *The Age,* 11 February 1997, p. B3.

7. S. Heath, "Mother's choice: being at home is 'more fulfilling,'" *The Age,* 4 April 1996, p. A15.

8. C. Hakim, "Labour mobility and employment stability: rhetoric and reality on the sex differential in labour market behavior," *European Sociological Review* 12 (1996): 45–69.

9. C. Hakim, "The sexual division of labour and women's heterogeneity," *British Journal of Sociology* 47, no. 1 (1996): 186.

10. G. Steinem, *Outrageous Acts and Everyday Rebellions,* second edition (New York: Henry Holt, 1995), p. 184.

11. B. Vobejda, "No maternal risk in day care: study," *The Age,* 22 April 1996, p. 1.

12. Kitzinger, *Ourselves as Mothers,* p. 28.

13. Brown, Lumley et al., *Missing Voices,* p. 165.

14. Ibid., p. 166.

15. D. Richardson, *Women, Motherhood and Childrearing* (London: Macmillan, 1993), p. 2.

16. J. Ribbens, *Mothers and Their Children: A Feminist Sociology of Childbearing* (London and Thousand Oaks, Calif.: Sage, 1994), p. 2.

17. C. Ford, "The hill of happiness," *The Age,* 11 February 1997, p. B3.

18. Heath, "Marriage, motherhood and other mayhem," p. B3.

19. M. Lowe and R. Hubbard, "Introduction," in *Woman's Nature: Rationalizations of Inequality* (New York: Pergamon Press, 1984), p. xi.

20. Ibid., p. x.

21. S. Ortner and H. Whitehead, "Introduction," in *Sexual Meanings: The Cultural Construction of Gender and Sexuality* (Cambridge, New York, and Melbourne: Cambridge University Press, 1981), p. 1.

22. Rowland, *Living Laboratories,* p. 7.

23. Birke, Himmelweit, and Vines, *Tomorrow's Child,* p. 18.

24. R. Winkler and M. van Keppel, *Relinquishing Mothers in Adoption: Their Long-term Adjustment* (Melbourne: Institute of Family Studies, May 1984), Monograph no. 3, p. 54.

25. Ibid., p. 1.

26. Quoted in S. Chick, *Searching for Charmian* (Sydney: Picador, 1994), p. 296.

27. Quoted in Claire, *The Abortion Dilemma*, p. 211.

28. M. Meggitt, untitled, in *Surrogacy—In Whose Interest? Proceedings of National Conference on Surrogacy,* The Mission of St. James and St. John, Melbourne, February 1991, p. 78.

29. E. Deykin et al., "The postadoption experience of surrendering parents," *American Journal of Orthopsychiatry* 54, no. 2 (1984): 272.

30. D. Kalmuss, P. Namerow, and U. Bauer, "Short-term consequences of parenting versus adoption among young unmarried women," *Journal of Marriage and the Family* 54 (February 1992), pp. 80–90.

31. F. Whitlock, "The diary of a bastard," *The Age,* 21 August 1991, p. 1.

32. Ibid., p. 1.

33. Hadley, *Abortion: Between Freedom and Necessity,* p. 48.

34. Rowland, "Introduction," in Kane, *Birth Mother,* p. xiii.

35. H. Dietrich, "Dissenting, views 2," *Surrogacy Report I,* The National Bioethical Consultative Committee, Commonwealth of Australia, 1990, p. 58.

36. F. Niles, "Every life is precious," *New Woman,* April 1996, p. 77.

37. Ginsburg, *Contested Lives,* pp. 109–10.

38. Ross, "Abortion and the death of the fetus," p. 241.

39. Quoted in Claire, *The Abortion Dilemma,* p. 69.

40. Quoted in Heath, "Marriage, motherhood and other mayhem," p. B3.

41. Matheson, "The abortion scam: pro-life's shocking new tactics," p. 76.

42. M. K. Blakely, "Hers," *The New York Times,* 9 April 1981, p. C2.

43. Clissa, "Unplanned pregnancy," p. 31.

44. Francke, *The Ambivalence of Abortion,* p. 7.

45. Clissa, "Unplanned pregnancy," p. 32.

46. Francke, *The Ambivalence of Abortion,* p. 4.

## Chapter 6. Rights, Responsibilities, and Killing from Care (pp. 127–136)

1. D. Callahan, "How technology is reframing the abortion debate," *Hastings Center Report,* February 1986, p. 41.

2. Ibid., p. 33.

3. D. Callahan, "An ethical challenge to prochoice advocates," *Commonweal,* 23 November 1990, p. 681.

4. Ibid., p. 41.

5. Petchesky, *Abortion and Woman's Choice,* p. 340.

6. P. Badham, "Christian belief and the ethics of in-vitro fertilization and abortion," *Bioethics News* (Monash University) 6, no. 2 (1987): 14.

7. Petchesky, *Abortion and Woman's Choice,* p. 272.

8. Ibid., p. 263.

9. Callahan, "How technology is reframing the abortion debate," p. 39.

10. "*Newsweek* poll: divisions and growing doubts," *Newsweek,* 14 January 1985, p. 22.
11. Callahan, "How technology is reframing the abortion debate," p. 33.
12. Personal communication.
13. Birke, Himmelweit, and Vines, *Tomorrow's Child,* pp. 289–90.

## Appendix (pp. 140–142)

1. See for instance K. Luker, *Abortion and the Politics of Motherhood* (Berkeley: University of California Press, 1984).
2. Ibid.
3. In reality it is unlikely that fetal evacuation will be as medically safe for women as current vacuum abortion methods. However, the scenario was shaped in this way in order to curtail certain areas of discussion.

# Bibliography

AAP. 1998. Womb donor hope. *The Age* (Melbourne), 25 May, 3.

AbouZahr, C. 1994. The epidemiology of unsafe abortion. *The Kangaroo* (December): 159–67.

Albury, R. (n.d.). Contesting technology, representing women: hard questions about activism. manuscript.

Alcoff, L., and E. Potter, eds. (1993). *Feminist Epistemologies*. Thinking Gender series. New York and London: Routledge.

Badham, P. 1987. Christian belief and the ethics of in-vitro fertilization and abortion. *Bioethics News* (Monash University) 6(2): 17–18.

Bernstein, I. M., M. Watson, et al. 1989. Maternal brain death and prolonged fetal survival. *Obstetrics & Gynecology* 74(3, pt. 2): 434–37.

Bertoia, C., and J. Drakich. (1993). The fathers' rights movement. *Journal of Family Issues* 14(4): 592–615.

Birke, L., S. Himmelweit, et al. 1990. *Tomorrow's Child: Reproductive Technologies in the 90s*. London: Virago.

Blakley, M. K. 1981. Hers. *New York Times*, 9 April. C2.

Bobejda, B. 1996. No maternal risk in day care: study. *The Age* (Melbourne), 22 April, 1.

Bowtell, E. 1995. Condoms, coitus and adolescents. *On the Level* 4(2): 14–19.

Boyce, N. 1998. Off the wall: wild ideas in medicine find a willing sponsor. *New Scientist* (11 April).

Brown, S., J. Lumley, et al. 1994. *Missing Voices: The Experience of Motherhood*. Melbourne: Oxford University Press.

Brownmiller, S. 1984. *Femininity*. New York: Fawcett Columbine.

Bruce, J. 1995. Reproductive choice: the responsibilities of men and women. *On the Level* 4(2): 26–27.

Bulletti, C. et al. 1988. Early human pregnancy in vitro utilizing an artificially perfused uterus. *Fertility and Sterility* 49(6): 991–96.

Callahan, D. 1986. How technology is reframing the abortion debate. *Hastings Center Report* (February): 33–42.

———. 1990. An ethical challenge to prochoice advocates. *Commonweal* (23 November), 681–87.

Cannold, L. 1994. Abortion pill hope. *The Age* (Melborne), 31 May. A18.

———. 1996. The new progestogen "third generation" oral contraceptive pills: how safe are they? *Healthsharing Women* 6(3–4): 14–18.

———. 1994. The ongoing debate about RU486. *Healthsharing Women* 5(2): 3–8.

———. 1997. "There is no evidence to suggest": changing the way we judge information for disclosure in the informed consent process. *Hypatia* 12(2): 165–84.

———. 1995. Women, ectogenesis and ethical theory. *Journal of Applied Philosophy* 12(1): 57–64.

———. 1996. A woman's sorrow. *The Age* (Melbourne), 1 November. 16.

Cannold, L., P. Singer, et al. 1996. What is the justice-care debate *really* about? *Midwest Studies in Philosophy* 20: 357–77.

Cannold-McDonald, L. 1992. Technical victory, political defeat. *The Age* (Melbourne), 8 July. 16.

Center for Reproductive Law and Policy. 1995. The status of a woman's right to choose. *Reproductive Freedom in the States*. 2.

Chick, S. 1994. *Searching for Charmian*. Sydney: Picador.

Churchill, L. S., J. J. Siman. 1982. Abortion and the rhetoric of individual rights. *The Hastings Center Report* 12(1): 9–12.

Claire, M. 1995. *The Abortion Dilemma: Personal Views on a Public Issue*. New York and London: Plenum.

Clissa, A. 1995. Unplanned pregnancy. *On the Level* 4(2): 28–33.

Concar, D. 1996. Into the mind of the unborn. *New Scientist*. 2052: 40–45.

Condit, C. M. 1990. *Decoding Abortion Rhetoric: Communicating Social Change*. Champaign: University of Illinois Press.

———. 1995. Fetal personhood: political identity under construction. In *Expecting Trouble: Surrogacy, Fetal Abuse and New Reproductive Technologies*. Edited by P. Boling. Boulder, Colo.: Westview Press.

Crouch, M., and L. Manderson. 1993. *New Motherhood: Cultural and Personal Transitions in the 1980s*. Amsterdam: Gordon and Breach Science Publishers.

Davies, J. A. 1997. New push on abortion pill. *The Sunday Age* (Melbourne), 18 May. 1.

Debelle, P. 1991. Ethics in embryo. *Good Weekend Magazine* (6 April): 18–22.

Deykin, E. et al. 1984. The postadoption experience of surrendering parents. *American Journal of Orthopsychiatry* 54(2): 271–80.

Dietrich, H. 1990. Dissenting views 2. Commonwealth of Australia, The National Bioethics Consultative Committee.

Dow, S. 1996. Technology of hope poses new dilemmas. *The Age* (Melbourne), 25 July. A13.

Dunne, R. 1990. Dissenting views 1. Commonwealth of Australia, The National Bioethics Consultative Committee.

Eisenberg, A., H. Murkoff, et al. 1993. *What to Expect When You're Expecting*. Sydney and Aukland: Angus & Robertson.

Elkins, T., H. Andersen, et al. 1989. Court-ordered cesarean section: an analysis of ethical concerns in compelling cases. *American Journal of Obstetrics and Gynecology* 161(1): 150–54.

Ewing, T. 1997. IVF breakthrough hailed. *The Age* (Melbourne), 2 May. 1.

Exactly what is partial birth abortion (PBA)? 1998. *Partial birth abortion protest.* World Wide Web, www.tidalweb.com/life/prolife.htm.

Fairweather, E. 1987. Abortion: the feelings behind the slogans. In *Women's Health: A Spare Rib Reader.* Edited by S. O'Sullivan. London: Pandora. 195–202.

Faludi, S. 1991. *Backlash: The Undeclared War against American Women.* New York: Crown.

Finlay, J. 1996. A fatal concern. *The Age* (Melbourne), 2 November. 23.

Ford, C. 1997. The hill of happiness. *The Age* (Melbourne), 11 February. B3.

Francke, L. 1978. *The Ambivalence of Abortion.* New York: Random House.

Gilligan, C. 1984. *In a Different Voice.* Cambridge and London: Harvard University Press.

Ginsburg, F. 1989. *Contested Lives: The Abortion Debate in an American Community.* Berkeley: University of California Press.

Gomberg, P. 1991. Abortion and the morality of nurturance. *Canadian Journal of Philosophy* 21(4): 513–24.

Grosz, E. 1993. Bodies and knowledges: feminism and the crisis of reason. In *Feminist Epistemologies.* Edited by L. P. Alcoff and E. Potter. New York and London: Routledge.

Grundmann, D. 1994. *Abortion after Twenty Weeks in Clinical Practice: Practical, Ethical and Legal Issues.* Ethical Issues in Prenatal Diagnosis and the Termination of Pregnancy, Melbourne, Centre for Human Bioethics.

Hadfield, P. 1992. Japanese pioneers raise kid in rubber womb. *New Scientist* (25 April): 5.

Hadley, J. 1996. *Abortion: Between Freedom and Necessity.* London: Vintage.

Hakim, C. 1996. Labour mobility and employment stability: rhetoric and reality on the sex differential in labour market behaviour. *European Sociological Review* 12: 45–69.

———. 1996. The sexual division of labour and women's heterogeneity. *British Journal of Sociology* 47(1): 178–88.

Handelsman, D. 1995. Male contraception: present and future. *On the Level* 4(2): 9–13.

Harding, S., and M. Hintikka, eds. 1983. *Discovering Reality: Feminist Perspectives on Epistemology, Metaphysics, and the Philosophy of Science.* Dordrecht: Reidel.

Harding, S. 1993. Rethinking standpoint epistemology: "What is strong objectivity." In *Feminist Epistemologies.* Edited by L. Alcoff and E. Potter. New York and London: Routledge.

Hartouni, V. 1997. *Cultural Conceptions: On Reproductive Technologies and the Remaking of Life.* Minneapolis and London: University of Minnesota Press.

Hartsock, N. 1983. The feminist standpoint: developing the ground for a specifically feminist historical materialism. In *Discovering Reality: Feminist Pespectives on Epistemology, Metaphysics, Methodolgy, and the*

*Philosophy of Science*. Edited by S. Harding and M. Hintikka. Dordrecht: Reidel.

Heath, S. 1996. Marriage, motherhood and other mayhem. *The Age* (Melbourne), 11 February. B3.

Hekman, S. 1997. Truth and method: feminist standpoint theory revisited. *Signs* 22(2): 341–65.

Held, V. 1993. *Feminist Morality: Transforming Culture, Society, and Politics*. Chicago and London: University of Chicago Press.

Henshaw, S., and K. Kost. 1996. Abortion patients in 1994–1995: characteristics and contraceptive use. *Family Planning Perspectives* 28(4): 1–16.

Hicks, K. 1994. *Surviving the Dalkon Shield IUD: Women v. the Pharmaceutical Industry*. New York and London: Teachers College Press.

Horsley, P., and S. Tremellin, eds. 1996. Old fights and new challenges: a roundtable discussion on abortion. *Healthsharing Women* (now *Women's Health Victoria*) 6 (June–September).

Jordon, B. 1993. *Birth in Four Cultures: A Crosscultural Investigation of Childbirth in Yucatan, Holland, Sweden, and the United States*. Prospect Heights, Illinois: Waveland.

Kalmuss, D., P. Namerow, et al. 1992. Short-term consequences of parenting versus adoption among young unmarried women. *Journal of Marriage and the Family* 54 (February): 80–90.

Kane, E. 1990. *Birth Mother*. Melbourne: Sun.

Karlin, E. 1995. An abortionist's credo. *Sunday New York Times*, 19 March. 32.

Kennison, K., and K. Hirsch. 1996. *Mothers: Twenty Stories of Contemporary Motherhood*. New York: North Point Press.

Kissane, K. 1995. Abortion doubts redefine debate. *The Age* (Melbourne), 25 October. 19.

Kitzinger, S. 1992. *Ourselves as Mothers*. Garden City: Doubleday.

Kolder, V., J. Gallagher, et al. 1987. Court-ordered obstetrical interventions. *The New England Journal of Medicine* 316(19): 1193–96.

Komesaroff, P., ed. 1995. *Troubled Bodies: Critical Perspectives on Postmodernism, Medical Ethics, and the Body*. Melbourne: Melbourne University Press.

Krutli, D. 1991. *Mid-trimester abortion service within a public hospital*. Women and Surgery, Melbourne, *Healthsharing Women* (now *Women's Health Victoria*).

Kulczycki, A., M. Potts, et al. 1996. Abortion and fertility regulation. *The Lancet* 347: 1663–68.

Lauritzen, P. 1997. Hear no evil, see no evil, think no evil: ethics and the appeal to experience. *Hypatia* 12(2): 83–104.

Lazzaro, J., J. Waugh, et al. 1991. Abortion an Act of Love: Sixteen Women Tell Their Stories. Melbourne: Melbourne University Social Enquiry and Social Work Research Project.

Lipsitch, M. 1993. The battle before birth. *The Age* (Melbourne), 9 August: 3.

Lowe, M., and R. Hubbard. 1984. *Women's Nature: Rationalizations of Inequality*. New York: Pergamon Press.

Lowinsky, N. 1992. *The Motherline: Every Woman's Journey to Find Her Female Roots*. Putnam's: New York.

Luker, K. 1975. *Abortion and the Decision Not to Contracept*. Berkeley: University of California Press.

———. 1984. *Abortion and the Politics of Motherhood*. Berkeley: University of California Press.

Mackenzie, C. 1995. Abortion and embodiment. In *Troubled Bodies: Critical Perspectives on Postmodernism, Medical Ethics, and the Body*. Edited by P. Komesaroff. Melbourne: Melbourne University Press.

Marsiglio, W. 1985. Husbands sex-role perferences and contraceptive intentions: the case of the male pill. *Sex Roles* 12(5–6): 655–63.

Matheson, A. 1996. The abortion scam: pro-life's shocking new tactics. *New Woman* (April): 74–162.

McDonnell, K. 1984. *Not an Easy Choice: A Feminist Re-examines Abortion*. Boston: South End Press.

Meggitt, M. 1991. *Untitled*. Submitted in the Conference: Surrogacy—In Whose Interest? From the proceedings of National Conference on Surrogacy. Published by The Mission of St. John and St. James, Melbourne.

Merleau-Ponty, M. 1962. *The Phenomenology of Perception*. New York: Humanities Press.

*Ms.* 1996. Call Iron John! *Ms.* 7: 27.

Neustatter, A., and G. Newson. 1986. *Mixed Feelings: The Experience of Abortion*. Sydney: Pluto Press.

Newman, K. 1996. *Fetal Positions: Individualism, Science, Visuality*. Stanford, Calif.: Stanford University Press.

*Newsweek*. 1985. *Newsweek* poll: divisions and growing doubts. *Newsweek* (14 January): 22.

NHMRC. 1996. *An information paper on termination of pregnancy in Australia*. Canberra, National Health and Medical Research Council.

———. 1995. *Services for the termination of pregnancy in Australia: a review*. Canberra, National Health and Medical Research Council.

Niles, F. 1996. Every life is precious. *New Woman* (April): 77.

Noonan, P. 1998. Abortion's children. *The Age*. (Melbourne). A29.

Oakley, A. 1987. From walking wombs to test-tube babies. In *Reproductive Technologies, Gender, Motherhood and Medicine*. Edited by M. Stanworth. Minneapolis: University of Minnesota Press. 57–80.

———. 1980. *Women Confined: Towards a Sociology of Childbirth*. New York: Schocken Books.

Ortner, S., and H. Whitehead. 1981. *Sexual Meanings: The Cultural Constructon of Gender and Sexuality*. Cambridge, New York, and Melbourne: Cambridge University Press.

Overall, C. 1987. *Ethics and Human Reproduction: A Feminist Analysis*. Boston: Allen & Unwin.

Petchesky, R. P. 1985. *Abortion and Woman's Choice: The State, Sexuality and Reproductive Freedom*. Boston: Northeastern University Press.

———. 1985. Abortion in the 1980s: feminist morality and women's health. In *Women, Health and Healing: Towards a New Perspective*. Edited by E. O. Levin and V. Olessen. New York: Tavistock.

————. 1987. Foetal images : the power of visual culture in the politics of reproduction. In *Reproductive Technologies, Gender, Motherhood and Medicine*. Edited by M. Stanworth. Minneapolis: University of Minnesota Press. 57–80.

Polatnick, R. 1996. Diversity in women's liberation ideology: how a black and white group of the 1960s viewed motherhood. *Signs* 21(3): 679–706.

Pollit, K. 1990. Fetal rights: a new assault on feminism. *The Nation*. (March): 26: 409–18.

Powell, S., and H. Stagoll. 1992. *When You Can't Have a Child*. Rozelle, North Sydney: Allen & Unwin.

Purdy, L. 1994. The baby in the body. *The Hastings Center Report* 24(1): 31–32.

*Reproductive Freedom News*. 1996. Canadian appeals court finds pregnant woman cannot be forced into drug treatment. New York: The Center for Reproductive Law and Policy. 16: 8.

————. 1996. Efforts to ban late abortion methods threaten *Roe v. Wade*. New York: The Center for Reproductive Law and Policy.

————. 1997. New York judge says dismissed anti-abortion nurses cannot sue hospital. New York: The Center for Reproductive Law and Policy. 13: 5.

————. 1998. Preliminary injuction issued against Virginia "partial-birth abortion" ban. New York: The Center for Reproductive Law and Policy. 11: 2.

————. 1996. South Carolina high court reinstates conviction for mother's behavior during pregnancy. New York: The Center for Reproductive Law and Policy. 13: 4.

————. 1996. Wisconsin court rules woman must stand trial for drinking during pregnancy. New York: The Center for Reproductive Law and Policy.

Rhoden, N. 1986. Trimesters and technology: revamping *Roe v. Wade*. *Yale Law Journal* 95: 639–97.

Ribbens, J. 1994. *Mothers and Their Children: A Feminist Sociology of Childbearing*. London and Thousand Oaks, California: Sage.

Rich, A. 1976. *Of Woman Born*. New York: Norton.

Richardson, D. 1993. *Women, Motherhood and Childrearing*. London: Macmillan.

Ross, S. 1982. Abortion and the death of the fetus. *Philosophy and Public Affairs* 2(3): 232–45.

Rothman, B. K. 1986. *The Tentative Pregnancy: Pre-natal Diagnosis and the Future for Motherhood*. New York: Viking.

Rowland, R. 1993. *Living Laboratories: Women and Reproductive Technology*. Sydney: Pan Macmillan.

Ryan, L., M. Ripper, et al. 1994. *We Women Decide*. South Australia, Women's Studies Unit, Faculty of Social Sciences, Flinders University.

Saigal, et al. 1991. Cognitive abilities and school performance of extremely low birth weight children and matched term control children at age 8 years. *The Journal of Pediatrics* 118: 751–60.

Singer, P., and D. Wells. 1984. *The Reproduction Revolution*. Oxford: Oxford University Press.

Singer, P., and H. Kuhse. 1985. *Should the Baby Live?: The Problem of Handicapped Infants*. Oxford: Oxford University Press.

Smart, C. 1989. *Feminism and the Power of the Law*. London: Routledge.

Smart, C., and S. Sevenhuijsen, eds. 1989. *Child Custody and Politics of Gender*. London: Routledge.

Smith, J. 1988. Abortion and moral development theory: listening with different ears. *International Philosophical Quarterly* 28(109): 31–51.

Spender, D. 1985. *Man Made Language*. London: Routledge & Kegan Paul.

Stanworth, M. 1987. Reproductive technologies: gender, motherhood and medicine. In *Reproductive Technologies, Gender, Motherhood and Medicine*. Edited by M. Stanworth. Minneapolis: University of Minnesota Press. 10–35.

Steinbock, B. 1992. *Life Before Birth: The Moral and Legal Status of Embryos and Fetuses*. New York and Oxford: Oxford University Press.

Steinem, G. 1995. *Outrageous Acts and Everyday Rebellions*. New York: Henry Holt.

Teplin, S. W. et al. 1991. Neurodevelopmental health and growth status at age 6 years of children with birth weights less than 1001 grams. *The Journal of Pediatrics* 118: 768–77.

The Boston Women's Health Collective. 1984. *The New Our Bodies, Ourselves*. New York: Simon & Schuster.

Thomson, J. J. 1986. A defence of abortion. In *Applied Ethics*. Edited by P. Singer. Oxford: Oxford University Press: 37–56.

Thornton, J. G., H. M. McNamara, et al. 1994. Would you rather be a "birth" or "genetic" mother: If so, how much? *Journal of Medical Ethics* 20(2): 87–92.

Vinzant, C. 1993. The ghastly inside story of how the rights-to-life movement stockpiles and uses aborted fetuses. *Spy* (May): 59–65.

Wallace, M. 1991. *Health Care and the Law: A Guide for Nurses*. North Ryde, N.S.W.: Law Book Company.

Watkins, S. 1998. 'Cavelier' abortionists slated by pro-life. *The Age* (Melbourne), 27 April. 6.

Wearing, B. 1984. *The Ideology of Motherhood: A Study of Sydney Suburban Mothers*. Sydney: Allen & Unwin.

Whitlock, F. 1991. The diary of a bastard. *The Age* (Melbourne), 21 August. 1–2.

Winkler, R., and M. van Keppel. 1984. *Relinquishing Mothers in Adoption: Their Long-term Adjustment*. Melbourne: Institute of Family Studies.

Wolf, N. 1995. Our bodies, our souls: rethinking pro-choice rhetoric. *The New Republic* (16 October): 26–35.

———. 1995. Staking a right to struggle. *The Age* (Melbourne), 25 October. 19.

Young, I. 1984. Pregnant embodiment: subjectivity and alienation. *The Journal of Medicine and Philosophy* 9: 45–62.

Zimmerman, M. K. 1977. *Passage Through Abortion*. New York: Praeger Special Studies.

# Index

About the Author

Leslie Cannold is a researcher and journalist currently working on a Ph.D. at the Department of Learning and Educational Development at The University of Melbourne. She holds a Master of Bioethics from the Centre of Human Bioethics at Monash University, where she studied under and worked with Professor Peter Singer. She was recently made an honorary fellow of the Centre for Philosophy and Public Issues at the University of Melbourne. She has published in a variety of mainstream, community-based, and academic journals.